A LAYERED DECLARATIVE APPROACH TO ONTOLOGY TRANSLATION WITH KNOWLEDGE PRESERVATION

Frontiers in Artificial Intelligence and Applications

Volume 116

Published in the subseries

Dissertations in Artificial Intelligence

Under the Editorship of the ECCAI Dissertation Board
Thesis Supervisor: Asunción Gómez-Pérez

Recently published in this series

Vol. 115. G. Phillips-Wren and L. Jain (Eds.), Intelligent Decision Support Systems in Agent-Mediated Environments
Vol. 114. A.C. Varzi and L. Vieu (Eds.), Formal Ontology in Information Systems – Proceedings of the Third International Conference (FOIS-2004)
Vol. 113. J. Vitrià et al. (Eds.), Recent Advances in Artificial Intelligence Research and Development
Vol. 112. W. Zhang and V. Sorge (Eds.), Distributed Constraint Problem Solving and Reasoning in Multi-Agent Systems
Vol. 111. H. Fujita and V. Gruhn (Eds.), New Trends in Software Methodologies, Tools and Techniques – Proceedings of the Third SoMeT_W04
Vol. 110. R. López de Mántaras and L. Saitta (Eds.), ECAI 2004 – Proceedings of the 16th European Conference on Artificial Intelligence
Vol. 109. E. Onaindia and S. Staab (Eds.), STAIRS 2004 – Proceedings of the Second Starting AI Researchers' Symposium
Vol. 108. V. Stefanuk and K. Kaijiri (Eds.), Knowledge-Based Software Engineering – Proceedings of the Sixth Joint Conference on Knowledge-Based Software Engineering
Vol. 107. F. Darses et al. (Eds.), Cooperative Systems Design – Scenario-Based Design of Collaborative Systems
Vol. 106. D. Bourcier (Ed.), Legal Knowledge and Information Systems – JURIX 2003: The Sixteenth Annual Conference
Vol. 105. Y. Kiyoki et al. (Eds.), Information Modelling and Knowledge Bases XV
Vol. 104. A. Abraham et al. (Eds.), Design and Application of Hybrid Intelligent Systems
Vol. 103. B. Tessem et al. (Eds.), Eighth Scandinavian Conference on Artificial Intelligence – SCAI'03
Vol. 102. C. Turchetti, Stochastic Models of Neural Networks
Vol. 101. G.L. Torres et al. (Eds.), Advances in Intelligent Systems and Robotics – LAPTEC'03
Vol. 100. I. Aguiló et al. (Eds.), Artificial Intelligence Research and Development
Vol. 99. D. Šuc, Machine Reconstruction of Human Control Strategies
Vol. 98. H. Fujita and P. Johannesson (Eds.), New Trends in Software Methodologies, Tools and Techniques – Proceedings of Lyee W_03: The Second International Workshop on Lyee Methodology
Vol. 97. H.U. Hoppe et al. (Eds.), Artificial Intelligence in Education – Shaping the Future of Learning through Intelligent Technologies
Vol. 96. S. Handschuh and S. Staab (Eds.), Annotation for the Semantic Web
Vol. 95. B. Omelayenko and M. Klein (Eds.), Knowledge Transformation for the Semantic Web
Vol. 94. H. Jaakkola et al. (Eds.), Information Modelling and Knowledge Bases XIV

ISSN 0922-6389

A Layered Declarative Approach to Ontology Translation with Knowledge Preservation

Oscar Corcho

Ontological Engineering Group, Departamento de Inteligencia Artificial, Universidad Politécnica de Madrid, Spain

IOS Press

Amsterdam • Berlin • Oxford • Tokyo • Washington, DC

ISBN 1 58603 477 4
Library of Congress Control Number: 2004116332

Publisher
IOS Press
Nieuwe Hemweg 6B
1013 BG Amsterdam
The Netherlands
fax: +31 20 620 3419
e-mail: order@iospress.nl

Distributor in the UK and Ireland
IOS Press/Lavis Marketing
73 Lime Walk
Headington
Oxford OX3 7AD
England
fax: +44 1865 750079

Distributor in the USA and Canada
IOS Press, Inc.
4502 Rachael Manor Drive
Fairfax, VA 22032
USA
fax: +1 703 323 3668
e-mail: iosbooks@iospress.com

PRINTED IN THE NETHERLANDS

Preface

Ontologies are widely used in the areas of Knowledge Engineering, Artificial Intelligence and Computer Science, in applications related to knowledge management, natural language processing, e-commerce, intelligent information integration, information retrieval, database design and integration, bio-informatics, education, and in new emerging fields like the Semantic Web and the Semantic Grid.

The word "Ontology" is taken from Philosophy, where it means a systematic explanation of being. It was in the last decade when ontologies became relevant as a solution to the knowledge acquisition bottleneck in the development of knowledge-based systems. Specifically, in 1991, it became extremely important when the DARPA Knowledge Sharing Effort [Neches et al., 1991, page 37] envisioned a new way to build knowledge-based systems, based on assembling reusable knowledge components instead of constructing new knowledge bases from scratch. With this new approach, systems would be able to share their declarative knowledge, modeled by means of ontologies, and their problem-solving techniques and reasoning services; and system developers would only need to worry about creating the specialized knowledge and reasoners new to the specific task of their system.

Since then, several definitions for the word "ontology" have been proposed in the literature, many of which are collected and explained in [Guarino and Giaretta, 1995] and [Gómez-Pérez et al., 2003]. One of the most cited definitions is proposed by Studer and colleagues [Studer et al., 1998], based on previous definitions of Gruber [Gruber, 1993a] and Borst [Borst, 1997]: "An ontology is a formal, explicit specification of a shared conceptualization". Conceptualization refers to an abstract model of some phenomenon in the world by having identified the relevant concepts of that phenomenon. Explicit means that the types of concepts used, and the constraints on their use are explicitly defined. Formal refers to the fact that the ontology should be machine-readable. Shared reflects the notion that an ontology captures consensual knowledge, that is, it is not the private opinion of some individual, but accepted by a group.

Ontologies can be implemented in varied ontology languages, which are usually divided in two groups: classical and ontology markup languages. Among the classical languages used for ontology construction we can cite (in alphabetical order): CycL [Lenat and Guha, 1990], FLogic [Kifer et al, 1995], KIF [Genesereth and Fikes, 1992], LOOM [MacGregor, 1991], OCML [Motta, 1999], and Ontolingua [Gruber, 1992]. Among the ontology markup languages, used in the context of the Semantic Web, we can cite: DAML+OIL [Horrocks and van Harmelen, 2001], OIL [Horrocks et al, 2000], OWL [Dean and Schreiber, 2004], RDF [Lassila and Swick, 1999], RDF Schema [Brickley and Guha, 2004], SHOE [Luke and Hefflin, 2000], and XOL [Karp et al, 1999]. Each of these languages has its own syntax, expressiveness, and reasoning capabilities, provided by different inference engines. Languages are also based on different knowledge representation paradigms or on combinations of them (frames, first order logic, description logic, semantic networks, topic maps, conceptual graphs, etc.).

A similar situation applies to ontology tools: several ontology editors and ontology management systems can be used to develop ontologies. Among them we can cite (in alphabetical order): KAON [Maedche et al., 2003], OilEd [Bechhofer et al., 2001], OntoEdit [Sure et al., 2002], the Ontolingua Server [Farquhar et al., 1997], OntoSaurus [Swartout et al., 1997], Protégé-2000 [Noy et al., 2000], WebODE [Arpírez et al., 2003], and WebOnto [Domingue, 1998]. As in the case of languages, the knowledge models underlying these tools have their own expressiveness and reasoning capabilities, since they are also based on different knowledge representation paradigms or on combinations of them. Besides, ontology tools usually export ontologies to one or several ontology languages and import ontologies coded in different ontology languages.

There are important connections and implications between the knowledge modeling components used to build an ontology in such languages and tools, and the knowledge representation paradigms used to formally represent such components. With frames and first order logic, the knowledge components commonly used to build ontologies are [Gruber, 1993a]: classes, relations, functions, formal axioms, and instances. With description logics, they are [Baader et al., 2003]: concepts, roles, and individuals. With semantic networks, they are: nodes and arcs between nodes.

The **ontology translation problem** [Gruber, 1993a] occurs when we decide to reuse an ontology (or part of an ontology) with a tool or language different from those in which the ontology is available. If ontology-based system developers are forced, individually, to commit to the task of translating and incorporating ontologies to their systems, they will require great time and effort to achieve their objectives [Swartout et al., 1997]. Therefore, ontology reuse in different contexts will be highly boosted as long as we provide ontology translation services between those languages and/or tools.

If we refer to the exchange of ontologies between ontology tools, the ontology translation problem is also known as the **interoperability problem**. In fact, interoperability is defined as "the ability of two or more systems or components to exchange information in a heterogeneous network and to use that information" [IEEE, 1999, page 2]. In the Ontological Engineering field, the term interoperability refers to the ability of different ontology tools to exchange their ontologies.

Many ontology translation systems can be found in the literature. They are mainly aimed at importing ontologies implemented in a specific ontology language to an ontology tool, or at exporting ontologies modeled with an ontology tool to an ontology language. A smaller number of ontology translation systems are aimed at transforming ontologies between ontology languages or between ontology tools.

Since ontology tools and languages have different expressiveness and reasoning capabilities, **translations between them are not straightforward nor easily reusable**. They normally require the making of many **decisions at different levels**, ranging from low layers (i.e., how to transform a concept name identifier from one format to another) to higher layers (i.e., how to transform a ternary relation among concepts to a format that only allows representing binary relations between concepts).

In this book we demonstrate that current ontology translation systems do not normally take into account such a layered structure of translation decisions. Also, in these systems **translation decisions are usually hidden inside their programming code**. Both aspects make it difficult to understand how ontology translation systems work.

In addition, the wide variety of expressiveness and reasoning capabilities of tools and languages makes it rather difficult to exchange ontologies between ontology languages and/or tools **without losing knowledge** from the original ontologies (aka, with semantic preservation) or **without changing their intended meaning** (aka, with pragmatic preservation). Achieving interoperability is difficult because not all the ontology components that can be represented in a source format can easily be transformed into a target one, and because not all the results of the transformations performed are easy to understand, either by human users or by software systems.

This book presents the results of my PhD thesis, which is focused on the ontology translation problem. This thesis has two main contributions to the state of the art:

- It proposes a new **model for building and maintaining ontology translation systems**, that is characterized by two main features. First, it identifies four layers where ontology translation decisions can be taken: lexical, syntax, semantic, and pragmatic. This **layered architecture** is based on existing work in formal languages and in the theory of signs (semiotics) [Morris, 1938]. Second, it proposes to represent ontology translation decisions **declaratively** in the language ODEDialect, which is composed of the languages ODELex, ODESyntax, and ODESem.
- It characterizes existing ontology translation approaches from the perspectives of **semantic and pragmatic preservation**, that is, consequence and intended meaning preservation, respectively. It also describes the lifecycle of ontologies in cyclic ontology translation processes, which are defined as successive translations where the initial source and final target formats coincide, and with one or more intermediate formats.

This book is structured as follows:

Chapter 1 (*State of the Art on Ontological Engineering*) presents a survey of the current state of ontology tools and languages, and how they have evolved during the last decades. We have especially focused on their similarities and differences, on their knowledge models and on their expressiveness and reasoning capabilities. The chapter also describes the current state of the art on ontology translation: we present the classifications of ontology translation problems proposed so far, different ontology translation architectures and the existing technology that supports them.

Chapter 2 (*Work Objectives*) describes the open research problems and goals, the contributions of this book to the state of the art, and the set of work assumptions, hypotheses, and restrictions considered in this work.

Chapter 3 (*A Layered Declarative Ontology Translation Model*) describes in detail the layered and declarative model proposed for building and maintaining ontology translation systems. In this model, ontology translation problems are divided into four layers – lexical, syntax, semantic, and pragmatic –, where different types of problems are dealt with. Besides, the model proposes to specify translation decisions at each layer by expressing declaratively how the different ontology components must be transformed from the source format into the target format. For this purpose, we propose to use the ODEDialect language, which is composed of three languages: ODELex, ODESyntax, and ODESem. Finally, the model proposes a method to follow when building ontology translation systems, taking into account the previous features.

Chapter 4 (*Semantic and Pragmatic Preservation in Ontology Translation*) presents the second contribution, namely how to preserve semantics and pragmatics in the ontology translation process. It analyses four proposals for ontology translation: indirect transformations that use common interchange formats; direct transformations that consist of establishing mappings between the knowledge models of the source and target formats;

direct transformations that use knowledge representation ontologies of the source and target formats; and direct transformations that combine direct mappings and knowledge representation ontologies. This chapter presents a comparison between these approaches with respect to their semantic and pragmatic preservation properties in cyclic transformations.

Chapter 5 (*Experimentation*) describes the experiments performed to evaluate the ontology translation model proposed: ontology translation systems from WebODE to RDF(S), OWL, and Protégé-2000, and vice versa. This chapter also describes the results obtained from using the ontology translation architectures proposed in Chapter 4 in the development of an ontology translation system between the tools WebODE and Protégé-2000: indirect transformations using KIF, RDF(S) and OWL as interchange languages, and the three types of direct ontology translations proposed.

Chapter 6 (*Conclusions and Future Work*) presents the main conclusions of this work, emphasizing its main contributions. The chapter also presents future work to be performed in the field of ontology translation.

The **appendix I** contains the BNF grammars of the three languages that compose ODEDialect: ODELex, ODESyntax, and ODESem.

Acknowledgements

I would like to thank Asunción Gómez-Pérez for her help and guidance during all these years. Since 1996, when we started working together, we have enjoyed deep discussions and long struggles about many aspects of the Ontological Engineering field. Besides, Asun has been always able to find a time slot in her extremely busy schedule to help me to structure the book contents, to read the early drafts of this document, and to propose many interesting improvements to it so as to make the ideas expressed here easier to understand.

I am also in debt to current and past members of the Ontological Engineering Group at UPM, with whom I have had many interesting discussions during my and their work and have shared many good moments. Among all of them, I would like to give special thanks to Mariano Fernández-López, who made so many helpful comments to improve this document, and who gave me important clues about knowledge representation ontologies and about different options for representing translators declaratively; to Rafael González-Cabero, who was in charge of implementing the RDF(S), DAML+OIL and OWL import services for the WebODE workbench and helped me to evaluate the ontology translation method described in Chapter 3; to Angel López-Cima, who has been patient enough to cope with my frequent programming errors in all the WebODE ontology translation systems developed; and to David Manzano, who made his large mathematical background available to me whenever I needed it.

I am particularly indebted to Rosario Plaza Arteche for her valuable help in checking and reviewing the grammar and spelling of the manuscript and improving its clarity and style, and to the members of the PhD thesis jury (Richard Benjamins, Daniel Borrajo, Jerome Euzenat, Ana García-Serrano, and Guus Schreiber), who provided very valuable comments that I have incorporated in this document.

Last but not least, I must thank my friends and family for believing in me, and understanding and helping me in my academic career. And among them, I want to thank Katy, for her love and support in everything I do, and for not complaining so much about my constant work during the last period of my thesis work.

The work described in this document has been supported by the European Commission in the context of the IST project Esperonto (IST-2001-34373).

List of Figures

List of Tables

Contents

Chapter 1
State of the Art on Ontological Engineering

This chapter presents a summary of the state of the art on Ontological Engineering that is relevant for ontology translation. Section 1.1 describes what an ontology is from the perspective of Computer Science. Section 1.2 deals with the modeling components normally used to define ontologies under different knowledge representation paradigms. Section 1.3 focuses on ontology languages: we show how they have evolved in the last decades, and which are the main similarities and differences between the most relevant ontology languages. Similarly, section 1.4 focuses on ontology tools: we explain how ontology tools have evolved, and we describe and compare their main features, focusing on their knowledge models and on the ontology languages that they are able to export to and to import from. Section 1.5 deals with the ontology translation problem: we present how translation problems have been classified in the literature, the translation architectures proposed so far and the technology available for building ontology translation systems between languages and/or tools. In section 1.6 we conclude with a summary of the main gaps in ontology translation and ontology tools interoperability in the current state of the art.

1.1 What is an Ontology?

As commented in the introduction, the word ontology is taken from Philosophy, where it means a systematic explanation of being. Whereas during the 1990s, this word became relevant for the Knowledge Engineering community. [Guarino and Giaretta, 1995] propose to use the words 'Ontology' (with the capital letter 'O') and 'ontology' to refer to the philosophical and Knowledge Engineering senses respectively. Many definitions about what an ontology is have been proposed in the literature. In this section, we will review these definitions and explain the relationships between them.

One of the first definitions was given by Neches and colleagues [Neches et al., 1991], who defined an ontology as follows:

> *An ontology defines the basic terms and relations comprising the vocabulary of a topic area as well as the rules for combining terms and relations to define extensions to the vocabulary.*

This descriptive definition gives some vague guidelines about what to do to build an ontology: identify basic terms and relations between terms, identify rules to combine terms, and provide the definitions of such terms and relations. Note that, according to Neches' definition, an ontology includes not only the terms that are explicitly defined in it but also the knowledge that can be inferred from it.

A few years later, Gruber [Gruber, 1993a] defined an ontology as follows:

An ontology is an explicit specification of a conceptualization.

This definition became the most quoted in literature and by the ontology community. Based on Gruber's definition, many definitions of what an ontology is were proposed. Borst [Borst, 1997] modified slightly Gruber's definition as follows:

Ontologies are defined as a formal specification of a shared conceptualization.

Then Gruber's and Borst's definitions were merged and explained by Studer and colleagues [Studer et al., 1998] as follows:

An ontology is a formal, explicit specification of a shared conceptualization. Conceptualization refers to an abstract model of some phenomenon in the world by having identified the relevant concepts of that phenomenon. Explicit means that the type of concepts used, and the constraints on their use are explicitly defined. Formal refers to the fact that the ontology should be machine-readable. Shared reflects the notion that an ontology captures consensual knowledge, that is, it is not private of some individual, but accepted by a group.

In 1995, Guarino and Giaretta [Guarino and Giaretta, 1995] collected and analyzed the following seven definitions:

1. *Ontology as a philosophical discipline.*
2. *Ontology as an informal conceptual system.*
3. *Ontology as a formal semantic account.*
4. *Ontology as a specification of a conceptualization.*
5. *Ontology as a representation of a conceptual system via a logical theory*
    - 5.1. *characterized by specific formal properties.*
    - 5.2. *characterized only by its specific purposes.*
6. *Ontology as the vocabulary used by a logical theory.*
7. *Ontology as a (meta-level) specification of a logical theory.*

On that paper, Guarino and Giaretta proposed to consider an ontology as:

A logical theory which gives an explicit, partial account of a conceptualization.

where a conceptualization is basically the idea of the world that a person or a group of people can have. Though on the surface the notion of conceptualization is quite similar to Studer and colleagues' notion, Guarino and Giaretta went a step further because they formalized the notion of conceptualization and established how to build the ontology by building a logical theory. Hence, strictly speaking, this definition would be only applicable to ontologies developed in logic. Guarino and Giaretta's was further refined in [Guarino, 1998], with the following definition:

A set of logical axioms designed to account for the intended meaning of a vocabulary.

There is another group of definitions based on the process to follow when building the ontology. These definitions also include some highlights about the relationship between ontologies and knowledge bases. For example, the definition given by Bernaras and colleagues [Bernaras et al., 1996] in the framework of the KACTUS project [Schreiber et al., 1995] is:

It [an ontology] provides the means for describing explicitly the conceptualization behind the knowledge represented in a knowledge base.

This definition proposes "extracting" the ontology from a knowledge base, what reflects the approach the authors use to build ontologies. In this approach, the ontology is built, following a bottom-up strategy, on the basis of an application knowledge base by means of an abstraction process. As more applications are built the ontology becomes more general, and, therefore, it moves further away from what would be a knowledge base.

Another strategy for building ontologies is to reuse large ontologies like SENSUS [Swartout et al., 1997] (with more than 70,000 nodes) to create domain specific ontologies and knowledge bases:

An ontology is a hierarchically structured set of terms for describing a domain that can be used as a skeletal foundation for a knowledge base.

According to this definition, the same ontology can be used for building several knowledge bases, which would share the same skeleton or taxonomy. Extensions of the skeleton should be possible at the low level by adding domain-specific subconcepts, or at the high level by adding intermediate or upper level concepts that cover new areas. If systems are built with the same ontology, they share a common underlying structure, therefore, merging and sharing their knowledge bases and inference mechanisms will become easier.

Sometimes the notion of ontology is diluted, in the sense that taxonomies are considered full ontologies [Studer et al., 1998]. For instance, UNSPSC[1], e-cl@ss[2], and RosettaNet[3], proposals for standards on the e-commerce domain, and the Yahoo! Directory, a taxonomy for searching the Web, are also considered ontologies [Lassila and McGuinness, 2001] because they provide a consensual conceptualization of a given domain. The ontology community distinguishes ontologies that are mainly taxonomies from ontologies that model the domain in a deeper way and provide *more restrictions* on domain semantics. The community calls them *lightweight* and *heavyweight ontologies* respectively. On the one hand, lightweight ontologies include concepts, concept taxonomies, relationships between concepts, and properties that describe concepts. On the other hand, heavyweight ontologies add axioms and constraints to lightweight ontologies. Axioms and constraints clarify the intended meaning of the terms gathered on the ontology.

Since ontologies are widely used for different purposes (natural language processing, knowledge management, e-commerce, intelligent integration of information, the Semantic Web, etc.) in different communities (i.e., knowledge engineering, databases and software engineering), Uschold and Jasper [Uschold and Jasper, 1999] provided a new definition of the word ontology to popularize it in other disciplines. Note that the database community as well as the object oriented design community also build domain models using concepts, relations, properties, etc., but most of the times they impose less semantic constraints than those imposed in heavyweight ontologies. Uschold and Jasper define an ontology as:

An ontology may take a variety of forms, but it will necessarily include a vocabulary of terms and some specification of their meaning. This includes definitions and an indication of how concepts are inter-related which collectively impose a structure on the domain and constrain the possible interpretations of terms.

---

[1] *http://www.unspsc.org/*
[2] *http://www.eclass.org/*
[3] *http://www.rosettanet.org/*

This section has gathered the most relevant definitions of the word ontology, which provide different and complementary points of view of the same reality. Some definitions are independent of the processes followed to build the ontology and of its use in applications, while others are influenced by its development process. The main conclusion to this section would be that ontologies aim to capture *consensual* knowledge in a generic way, and that they may be reused and shared across software applications and by groups of people. They are usually built cooperatively by different groups of people in different locations.

1.2 Which are the Main Components of an Ontology?

Heavyweight and lightweight ontologies can be modeled with different knowledge modeling techniques and they can be implemented in various kinds of languages [Uschold and Grüninger, 1996]. Ontologies can be *highly informal* if they are expressed in natural language; *semi-informal* if expressed in a restricted and structured form of natural language; *semi-formal* if in an artificial and formally defined language (i.e., Ontolingua [Farquhar et al., 1997], OWL [Dean and Schreiber, 2004]); and *rigorously formal* if they provide meticulously defined terms with formal semantics, theorems and proofs of properties such as soundness and completeness[4]. According to the definition of [Studer et al., 1998], a highly informal ontology would not be an ontology since it is not machine-readable.

There are important connections and implications between the knowledge modeling components (concepts, roles, etc.) used to build an ontology, the knowledge representation (KR) paradigms (frames, description logic, first order logic) used to represent formally such components, and the languages used to implement the ontologies in a given KR paradigm.

This section presents different techniques that could be applied to model ontologies. Not all of them can represent the same knowledge with the same degree of formality and granularity. The section describes which components are used to model heavyweight ontologies with AI-based approaches that combine frames and first order logic or use description logic, and points out which other techniques could also be used to model lightweight ontologies.

1.2.1 Modeling Heavyweight Ontologies with Frames and First Order Logic

[Gruber, 1993a] proposed to model ontologies using frames and first order logic. He identified five kinds of components: classes, relations, functions, formal axioms, and instances.

Classes represent concepts, which are taken in a broad sense, that is, they can represent abstract concepts (intentions, beliefs, feelings, etc.) or specific concepts (people, computers, tables, etc.). Classes in the ontology are usually organized in taxonomies through which inheritance mechanisms can be applied.

In the frame-based KR paradigm, metaclasses can also be defined. Metaclasses are classes whose instances are classes. They usually allow for gradations of meaning, since they establish different layers of classes in the ontology where they are defined.

Relations represent a type of association between concepts of the domain. They are formally defined as any subset of a product of n sets, that is: $R \subset C1 \times C2 \times ... \times Cn$. In the

[4] *Inspired by classical first order logic terminology (Hermes, 1973) (Lloyd, 1993), an ontology is sound if and only if it does not allow deducing invalid conclusions. An ontology is complete if and only if it allows deducing all the possible valid conclusions starting from the ontology vocabulary and applying the deduction rules permitted.*

case of binary relations, the first argument is known as the domain of the relation, and the second is the range. For instance, the binary relation *Subclass-Of* is used for building the class taxonomy.

Relations can be also domain dependent, expressing relationships between the instances of two concepts of a specific domain. Binary relations are sometimes used to express concept attributes (aka slots). Attributes are usually distinguished from relations because their range is a datatype, such as *string*, *number*, etc., while the range of relations is a concept.

Functions are a special case of relations in which the *n-th* element of the relation is unique for the *n-1* preceding elements. This is usually expressed as: F: C1 x C2 x ... x Cn-1 → Cn.

According to Gruber, ***formal axioms*** serve to model sentences that are always true. They are normally used to represent knowledge that cannot be formally defined by the other components. In addition, formal axioms are used to verify the consistency of the ontology itself or the consistency of the knowledge stored in a knowledge base.

Finally, ***instances*** are used to represent elements or individuals in an ontology.

1.2.2 Modeling Heavyweight Ontologies with Description Logic

Description Logic[5] (DL) is a logical formalism whose first implementation languages and systems were, as will be described in section 1.3, the following: KL-ONE [Brachman and Schmolze, 1985], Krypton [Brachman et al., 1983], Classic [Borgida et al., 1989], LOOM [MacGregor, 1991] and Kris [Baader and Hollunder, 1991]. Description Logic theories are divided into two parts: the TBox and the ABox. The TBox contains intensional (terminological) knowledge in the form of a terminology and describes general properties of concepts. The ABox contains extensional (assertional) knowledge, which is specific to the individuals of the discourse domain [Baader et al., 2003]. In other words, the TBox contains the definitions of concepts and roles, while the ABox contains the definitions of individuals (instances).

Basically, in DL systems we represent ontologies with three kinds of components: concepts, roles and individuals. ***Concepts*** in DL have the same meaning as in the frame paradigm: they represent classes of objects. ***Roles*** describe binary relations between concepts, hence they also allow the description of properties of concepts. Higher arity relations among concepts are also allowed in some DL languages and systems. Finally, ***individuals*** represent instances of classes.

Concepts and roles are both described with terminological descriptions, which are built from pre-existing terms and with a set of constructors (conjunction, disjunction, negation, value restriction, existential quantification, existential restriction, qualified number restriction, etc.). The choice and combination of the different constructors permit designing different DL languages, as shown in table 1.1. For example, a SHIQ language is a language that combines (ALC_{R+}) intersection, value restriction, limited existential quantification, the concepts *top* and *bottom*, atomic negation, negation, union, existential restriction, and transitive roles; with (H) role hierarchies; (I) inverse roles; and (Q) qualified number restrictions. The different combinations of constructors give different expressiveness/reasoning tradeoffs to the corresponding language [Baader et al., 2003].

Concepts in DL can be *primitive* (if they are defined specifying necessary conditions for the individuals of that concept) or *defined* (if they are defined specifying both necessary and sufficient conditions that must be satisfied by individuals of the concept).

---

[5] *Names previously used for Description Logic were: terminological knowledge representation languages, concept languages, term subsumption languages, and KL-ONE-based knowledge representation languages.*

Table 1.1. Common DL constructors and their correspondence with language names[6].

<table>
<tr><th>Construct</th><th>Syntax</th><th colspan="4">Language</th></tr>
<tr><td>Concept</td><td>A</td><td rowspan="4">FL_0</td><td rowspan="7">FL^-</td><td rowspan="8">AL</td><td rowspan="11">S[7]</td></tr>
<tr><td>Role name</td><td>R</td></tr>
<tr><td>Intersection</td><td>$C \cap D$</td></tr>
<tr><td>Value restriction</td><td>$\forall R.C$</td></tr>
<tr><td>Limited existential quantification</td><td>$\exists R$</td><td rowspan="3"></td></tr>
<tr><td>Top or Universal</td><td>$\top$</td></tr>
<tr><td>Bottom</td><td>$\bot$</td></tr>
<tr><td>Atomic negation</td><td>$\neg A$</td><td colspan="2"></td></tr>
<tr><td>Negation[8]</td><td>$\neg C$</td><td colspan="3">C</td></tr>
<tr><td>Union</td><td>$C \cup D$</td><td colspan="3">U</td></tr>
<tr><td>Existential restriction</td><td>$\exists R.C$</td><td colspan="3">E</td></tr>
<tr><td>Number restrictions</td><td>$(\geq n R)$ $(\leq n R)$</td><td colspan="3">N</td><td></td></tr>
<tr><td>Nominals</td><td>$\{a_1 \dots a_n\}$</td><td colspan="3">O</td><td></td></tr>
<tr><td>Role hierarchy</td><td>$R \subseteq S$</td><td colspan="3">H</td><td></td></tr>
<tr><td>Inverse role</td><td>R^-</td><td colspan="3">I</td><td></td></tr>
<tr><td>Qualified number restriction</td><td>$(\geq n R.C)$ $(\leq n R.C)$</td><td colspan="3">Q</td><td></td></tr>
</table>

Roles in DL can be either primitive or defined (also called derived). Many DL systems do not permit defining derived roles, because of their reasoning disadvantages, though they do permit the creation of role hierarchies. Regarding n-ary roles, some DL systems do not permit defining them, but only binary ones.

Formal axioms in DL use a subset of the constructs of first order logic. They are usually embedded in concept or role definitions.

Individuals represent instances of concepts and the values of their roles (properties). DL systems usually separate descriptions of individuals from concept and role descriptions. The former are included in the ABox (assertional knowledge) while the latter are included in the TBox (terminological knowledge)[9].

The last comment about DL is on the reasoning capabilities of this paradigm. The decision about which constructs to use in a DL language has strong effects not only on its expressiveness, but also on its reasoning power. Reasoning in DL is mainly based on concept subsumption, for which DL systems provide efficient automatic classifiers. From subsumption tests, DL systems derive concept satisfiability and consistency in the models represented. These classifiers are commonly built by means of tableaux calculus and constraint systems.

1.2.3 Modeling Lightweight Ontologies with Software Engineering and Database Modeling Techniques

Other techniques widely used in software engineering and databases for modeling concepts, relationships between concepts, and concept attributes, such as Entity-Relationship diagrams or UML class diagrams, could also be appropriate for building lightweight

[6] *In this table, we use A to refer to atomic concepts (concepts that are the basis for building other concepts), C and D to any concept definition, R to atomic roles and S to role definitions. FL is used for structural DL languages and AL for attributive languages [Baader et al., 2003].*

[7] *S is the name used for the language ALC_{R+}, which is composed of ALC plus transitive roles.*

[8] *ALC and ALCUE are equivalent languages, since union (U) and existential restriction (E) can be represented using negation (C).*

[9] *In some DL systems, the ABox also contains rules that allow inferring information. Some discussions have arisen about whether rules should be defined in the TBox or in the Abox. We think rules should be placed in the TBox, as they really define intensional rather than assertional knowledge.*

ontologies. These techniques impose a structure to the domain knowledge and constrain the interpretations of terms.

However, it is important to remark that the model can only be considered an ontology if it is a shared and consensual knowledge model agreed by a community. The use of these techniques for building lightweight ontologies is described in [Gómez-Pérez et al., 2003; chapter 1].

1.3 Ontology Languages

Several ontology languages have been created during the last decades and other general Knowledge Representation (KR) languages and systems have been used for implementing ontologies though these were not specifically created for this purpose. In this section we first explain how the most representative ontology languages have evolved in this period. Then we describe different formal and informal approaches used to compare their representation and/or reasoning capabilities. Finally, we compare those languages using an informal approach, which has been used successfully for determining the language or languages that best fit the representation and reasoning needs of several ontology-based applications.

1.3.1 Ontology Language Evolution

At the beginning of the 1990s, a set of AI-based ontology languages was created. Basically, the KR paradigms underlying such ontology languages were based on first order logic (e.g., KIF), on frames combined with first order logic (e.g., CycL, Ontolingua, OCML and FLogic), and on description logic (e.g., LOOM). OKBC was also created as a protocol to access ontologies implemented in different languages with a frame-based KR paradigm. The overall layout of these languages is shown in figure 1.1.

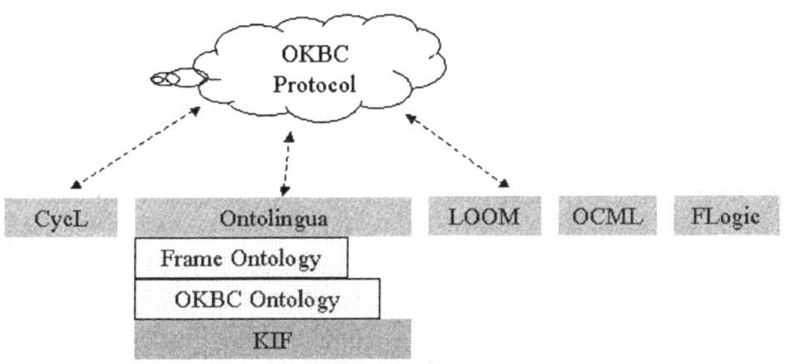

Figure 1.1. Overview of traditional ontology languages.

Of the previous set of languages, **CycL** [Lenat and Guha, 1990] was the first to be created. CycL is based on frames and first order logic and was used for building the Cyc Ontology.

KIF [Genesereth and Fikes, 1992][NCITS, 1998] was created later, in 1992, and was designed as a knowledge interchange format; KIF is based on first order logic, with some extensions to deal with sets, numbers, etc. Since ontologies were difficult to create directly in KIF, **Ontolingua** [Farquhar et al., 1997] was created on top of it. Ontolingua has a Lisp-like syntax and its underlying knowledge representation (KR) paradigm are frames and first order logic. Ontolingua was considered a standard *de facto* by the ontology community in the 1990s.

LOOM [MacGregor, 1991] was built at the same time, though it was not intended to implement ontologies but to create general knowledge bases. LOOM is based on description logic (DL) and production rules and provides automatic concept classification features. **OCML** [Motta, 1999] was developed later, in 1993, as a kind of "operational Ontolingua". In fact, most of the definitions that can be expressed in OCML are similar to the corresponding definitions in Ontolingua. OCML was built for developing executable ontologies and models in problem solving methods (PSMs). Finally, in 1995 **FLogic** [Kifer et al., 1995] was released (although its development started several years before) as a language that combined frames and first order logic though it did not have Lisp-like syntax.

In the spring of 1997, the High Performance Knowledge Base program (HPKB)[10] was started. This research program was sponsored by DARPA and its objective was to solve many of the problems that usually appear when dealing with large knowledge bases (concerning efficiency, content creation, integration of the content available in different systems, etc.). One of the results of this program was the development of the **OKBC** (Open Knowledge Base Connectivity) protocol [Chaudhri et al., 1998]. This protocol allows accessing knowledge bases stored in different Knowledge Representation Systems, which may be based on different KR paradigms. Of the languages aforementioned Ontolingua, LOOM and CycL are OKBC compliant.

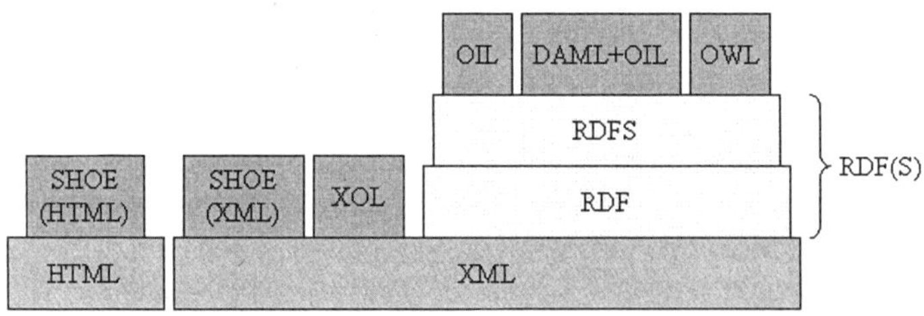

Figure 1.2. Ontology markup languages.

The boom of the Internet led to the creation of ontology languages for exploiting the characteristics of the Web. Such languages are usually called *web-based ontology languages* or *ontology markup languages*. Their syntax is based on existing markup languages such as HTML [Raggett et al., 1999] and XML [Bray et al., 2000], whose purpose is not ontology development but data presentation and data exchange respectively. The relationships between these languages are shown in figure 1.2.

The first ontology markup language appeared in 1996. This language was **SHOE** [Luke and Heflin, 2000]. SHOE is a language that combines frames and rules. It was built as an extension of HTML. It used tags different than those of the HTML specification, thus allowing the insertion of ontologies in HTML documents. Later its syntax was adapted to XML.

The rest of ontology markup languages are based on XML. **XOL** [Karp et al., 1999] was developed as a XMLization of OKBC-Lite, a small subset of primitives from the OKBC protocol. **RDF** [Lassila and Swick, 1999] was developed by the W3C (the World Wide Web Consortium) as a semantic-network based language to describe Web resources. Its development started in 1997, and RDF was proposed as a W3C Recommendation in 1999. The **RDF Schema** [Brickley and Guha, 2004] language was also built by the W3C as an extension to RDF with frame-based primitives. This language was first proposed as a W3C Candidate Recommendation in 2000 and then it suffered a major revision in November 2002, so that its reference document was published as a W3C Working Draft. Finally, it was proposed as a W3C Recommendation in February 2004. The combination of both RDF and RDF Schema is normally known as **RDF(S)**.

[10] *http://reliant.teknowledge.com/HPKB/*

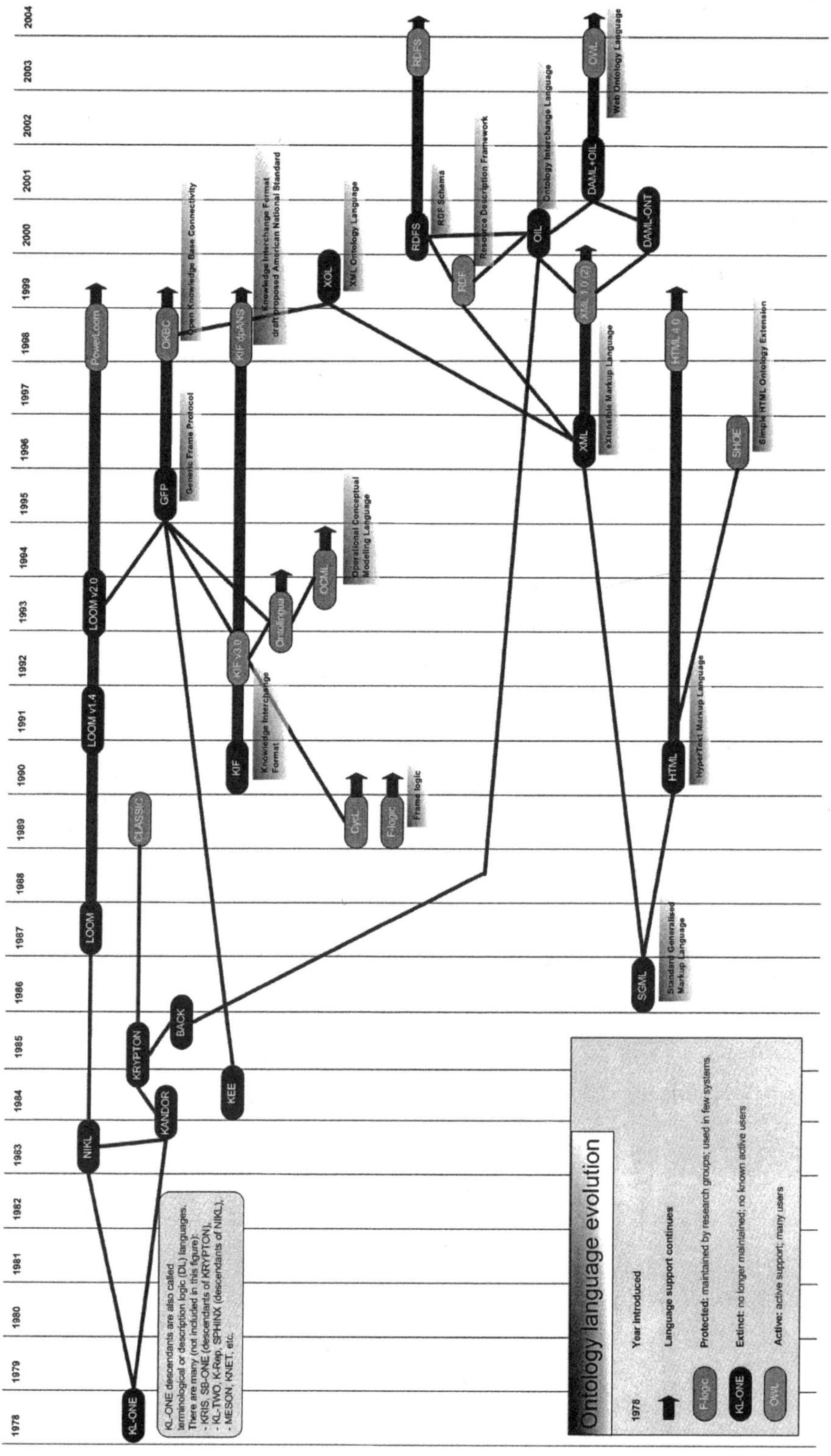

Figure 1.3: Ontology language evolution

These languages have established the foundations of the Semantic Web [Berners-Lee, 1999]. In this context three more languages have been developed as extensions to RDF(S): OIL, DAML+OIL, and OWL. **OIL** [Horrocks et al., 2000] was developed at the beginning of the year 2000 in the framework of the European IST project On-To-Knowledge[11]. It adds frame-based KR primitives to RDF(S) and its formal semantics is based on description logic. **DAML+OIL** [Horrocks and van Harmelen, 2001] was created later (between the years 2000 and 2001) by a joint committee from the US and the EU in the context of the DARPA project DAML[12]. It was based on the previous DAML-ONT language, built at the end of 2000, and on OIL. DAML+OIL adds DL-based KR primitives to RDF(S). In 2001 the W3C formed a working group called Web-Ontology (WebOnt) Working Group[13]. The aim of this group was to make a new ontology markup language for the Semantic Web. The result of their work is the **OWL** language [Dean and Schreiber, 2004], which is a W3C Recommendation (February 2004). OWL covers most of the features of DAML+OIL and has renamed most of the primitives that appeared in that language.

Figure 1.3 shows how these languages have evolved, and it also shows the relationships of these languages with other existing KR languages and systems.

1.3.2 KR Language Comparison Frameworks

Not all of the existing languages have the same expressiveness nor do they reason the same way. KR paradigms underlying ontology languages are diverse: frames, description logic, first (and second) order logic, semantic networks, etc.; besides some languages combine more than one KR paradigm. This fact makes very important to make an appropriate selection of the implementation language of an ontology. In fact, a KR paradigm may prove to be appropriate for a specific task but not for others carried out in an application.

Consequently, before coding an ontology the ontology developer should detect first what is needed in terms of expressiveness and reasoning, and then which languages satisfy such requirements. Several formal and informal approaches have been proposed to compare KR languages and systems. These approaches usually distinguish two dimensions –knowledge representation and reasoning mechanisms– and deal with features from one or both of them.

1.3.2.1 Formal Approaches for KR Language Comparison

According to the theory of signs (aka semiotics) [Morris, 1938], there are three aspects to be considered in the formal study of a language and of communication:

- Syntax: it deals with how symbols are structured.
- Semantic: it deals with what symbols mean.
- Pragmatic: it deals with how symbols are interpreted or used, considering features such as the environment and the mental state of the agents involved in a communication, which are external to the language.

The three aspects are tightly interrelated, although the meaning of a communication is, intuitively, a combination of the two latter aspects: semantic and pragmatic.

Existing formal approaches for KR language comparison are mainly focused on the semantic aspect of languages. They are normally used to prove that certain expressions in a language can or cannot be expressed in another. Therefore they allow measuring to a

---

[11] *http://www.ontoknowledge.org/*
[12] *http://www.daml.org/*
[13] *http://www.w3.org/2001/sw/WebOnt/*

certain extent the amount of knowledge that would be lost and preserved in the translation process between languages[14]. Basically, the following three approaches can be distinguished:

[Baader, 1996] proposes to define formally the expressive power of a language by means of the language semantics, which can be determined with different techniques such as model theory or axiomatic semantics. Once the semantics of two languages are determined, it is possible to analyze whether they have the same expressive power or not. Two languages have the ***same expressive power*** if they share the same models, taking into account the following two translation functions:

- ψ:Pred(Γ_1)→Pred(Γ_2), which transforms the predicates of the source language into the target language, creating any auxiliary predicates needed in the translation process.
- χ:L_1→L_2, which transforms any expression of the source language into the target language.

Similarly, [Borgida, 1996] defines the ***same expressiveness***[15] relation as follows: the language L_2 is as expressive as the language L_1 if there is a total function *transl*:L_1→L_2 such that for every sentence L in L_1, *transl*(L) expresses the meaning of L in L_2. The meaning of formulae is obtained by means of an interpretation function, as it is usually done in first order logic.

[Euzenat and Stuckenschmidt, 2001] and [Stuckenschmidt, 2003] define formally the ***coverage relation*** between languages as a relation that holds between L_1 and L_2 whenever there exists a mapping τ:L_1→L_2 that transforms every expression of L_1 into an expression of L_2. We should notice here the difference with respect to the previous definitions: the existence of a translation function is enough to determine that a language covers another, without considering whether the transformation preserves the semantics or not.

These formal approaches are useful to determine whether an expression in a language can be expressed in another language or not, by giving a formal proof of the transformation to be performed. However, they are time-consuming if we want to determine whether all the expressions of a language can be expressed in another, and they do not specify how the translation function has to be created. Only the latter approach has been used in ontology translation, with the aim of determining the transformation preservation properties of ontology translation systems in families of ontology languages, as described in section 1.5.

Moreover, these approaches require that the languages to be compared have formal semantics. Some KR languages and most of the ontology tools' knowledge models lack from formal semantics (e.g., OKBC, SHOE, XOL, OntoEdit, Protégé-2000, WebODE, etc.). This lack of formal semantics is a source of confusion and misunderstanding, and therefore it makes their formal comparison impossible [Hayes, 1974].

1.3.2.2 Semi-formal and Informal Approaches for KR Language Comparison

To overcome the difficulties of the aforementioned formal approaches, several complementary semi-formal and informal approaches have been proposed to show the similarities and differences of the knowledge models of ontology languages and tools.

[Corcho and Gómez-Pérez, 2000] proposed the first semi-formal comparison approach, which consists in a comparison framework of the expressiveness and reasoning capabilities

---

[14] *Similarly, these approaches can be applied to the comparison of the knowledge models of ontology tools.*

[15] *Different authors use different terms to refer to the fact that two languages can express the same knowledge: same expressive power, same expressiveness, and language coverage.*

of ontology languages based on the ontology components most commonly used in frame-based systems and on the reasoning mechanisms commonly present in ontology languages. The advantages of this approach is that it gives at a glance a coarse-grained comparison of languages that helps in finding their main similarities and differences. The main features that are compared in this framework for each dimension are described below:

With respect to the knowledge representation (language expressiveness) dimension, the framework deals with **concepts** and their **attributes**. It distinguishes two types of attributes: *instance attributes* (which describe concept instances and take values in them) and *class attributes* (which describe concepts and take values in them). The framework also deals with how attributes can be constrained according to their *type of value*, *cardinalities* (how many values the attribute can take), and other constraints such as the addition of procedural knowledge. It also shows whether the language allows representing metaclasses or not.

The framework also covers concept **taxonomies**. It analyses whether a language allows expressing subclass-of relationships, disjoint and exhaustive decompositions and partitions.

Relations are very important components in ontology modeling as they describe the relationships that can be established between concepts and between the instances of those concepts. They are usually called *relations* or *slots* in frame-based languages and *roles* or *properties* in DL-based languages. The framework analyses whether the language allows expressing binary and n-ary relations, relation hierarchies and general integrity constraints of relations.

The framework also deals with **functions**, if they can be defined in the language.

Finally, it deals with other ontology components, such as **formal axioms**, which represent sentences that are always true, and which are normally used to represent general restrictions of the domain or pieces of knowledge that cannot be implemented in the ontology with the rest of modeling components. Other components dealt with by the framework are **instances**, **rules**, **procedures**, etc.

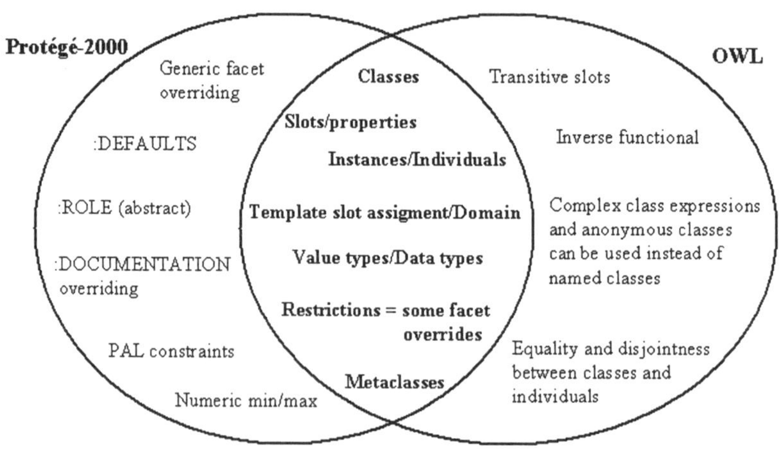

Figure 1.4. Informal comparison of the knowledge models of Protégé-2000 and OWL, using Venn diagrams [Knublauch, 2003].

With respect to the reasoning dimension, the framework deals with several aspects that can be found in their associated inference engines, such as the availability of **automatic classifiers** that compute the concept taxonomy automatically from the ontology concept definitions, the management of **simple** and/or **multiple inheritance** of concept attributes and relations through concept taxonomies, the management of **exceptions** in concept taxonomies (this is also called non-monotonic reasoning), and other **constraint checking** functionalities for detecting inconsistencies in the ontology.

The are other less formal comparison approaches. For instance, figure 1.4 shows the result of applying an informal comparison approach to compare the knowledge models of Protégé-2000 and OWL [Knublauch, 2003]. This approach uses Venn diagrams to show which components can be defined in both formats, and which ones are specific of each format. From the figure, it can be inferred that classes, slots, instances, etc., can be defined in both formats (although they have in some cases different names, such as slots for Protégé-2000 and properties for OWL); that default values, PAL constraints, etc., can be defined in Protégé-2000 but not in OWL; and that transitive slots, disjointness between classes, etc., can be defined in OWL but not in Protégé-2000.

1.3.3 Comparison of Ontology Languages

Table 1.2 shows the results of comparing the expressiveness of the most relevant ontology languages with the aforementioned semi-formal comparison approach. This study does not aim to show an exhaustive list of features of all these languages since each of them is based on different KR paradigms and has its own distinguishing features. Nor does it aim to establish a score of languages (in the sense of "language L_1 is better than language L_2"), since different, and sometimes incompatible, features may be needed for different ontology-based applications. It mainly aims to help understand better the similarities and differences between these languages.

The cells in the table are filled with '+' to indicate that it is a supported feature in the language; with '-' for non supported features; and with 'W' for non supported features that could be supported with some workaround. Examples of such workarounds are described in [Gómez-Pérez et al., 2003], and extended versions of this study can be found in [Corcho and Gómez-Pérez, 2000] and [Gómez-Pérez and Corcho, 2002].

The analysis of the table reveals the different expressive power of each language. There are relevant differences in expressiveness between traditional languages and ontology markup languages. While some languages permit representing heavyweight ontologies (with formal axioms, functions, rules, procedures, and other rich modeling components), others only permit representing lightweight ontologies (concepts, concept taxonomies, and relations between them). In fact, most of the modeling components can be represented in traditional languages (such as Ontolingua, LOOM and OCML), while ontology markup languages do not normally provide the means to represent all of them.

The following comments can be made on each of the main features presented in the table.

The table shows that **metaclasses** can be created in half of the languages. OWL DL does not allow defining metaclasses, but OWL Full allows them. As described in chapter 4, metaclasses can be useful for some of the translation approaches proposed.

All the ontology languages allow representing concepts and their **attributes** (aka slots, roles, and properties). Instance attributes can be defined in all the languages, and class attributes cannot be represented them in SHOE, RDF(S), and in none of the DL-based languages (LOOM, OIL, DAML+OIL, and OWL DL). This is due to the fact that reasoning with these attributes in description logic is difficult. However, class attributes can be represented in RDF(S), DAML+OIL, and OWL (which becomes OWL Full) with a workaround, as specified in the table. This workaround consists in defining class attributes as properties whose domain is the class *rdfs:Class*, *daml:Class*, and *owl:Class* respectively, and specifying their value(s) in the concept definition where the class attribute takes a value.

Table 1.2. Semi-formal comparison of ontology language expressiveness.

	Ontolingua	LOOM	OKBC	OCML	FLogic	SHOE	XOL	RDF(S)	OIL	DAML+OIL	OWL DL
CONCEPTS	+	+	+	+	+	+	+	+	+	+	+
Metaclasses	+	-	+	+	-	-	-	+	-	+	-
Attributes											
Instance attributes	+	+	+	+	+	+	+	+	+	+	+
Class attributes	+	-	+	+	+	-	+	W	-	W	W
Facets											
Type constraints	+	+	+	+	+	+	+	+	+	+	+
Cardinality constraints	+	+	+	+	W	-	+	-	+	+	+
Procedural knowledge	-	+	-	+	-	-	-	-	-	-	-
CONCEPT TAXONOMIES											
Subclass-Of	+	+	+	+	+	+	+	+	+	+	+
Disjoint-Decomposition	+	+	-	+	W	-	-	-	+	+	+
Exhaustive-Decomposition	+	-	-	W	W	-	-	-	W	W	W
Partition	+	+	-	+	W	-	-	-	+	+	W
RELATIONS											
Binary relations	+	+	+	+	+	+	+	+	+	+	+
n-ary relations	+	+	W	+	W	+	W	W	W	W	W
Relation hierarchies	+	+	-	+	W	-	-	+	+	+	+
Integrity constraints	+	+	-	+	+	-	-	-	-	-	-
FUNCTIONS											
Binary functions	+	+	W	+	+	-	W	-	+	+	+
n-ary functions	+	+	-	+	+	-	-	-	-	-	-
OTHER COMPONENTS											
Instances	+	+	+	+	+	+	+	+	+	+	+
Formal Axioms	+	+	-	+	+	-	-	-	-	-	-
Rules	-	+	-	+	-	+	-	-	-	-	-
Procedures	I	+	-	+	-	-	-	-	-	-	-

If we deal with **facets** (attribute constraints), we can see that all languages allow constraining the type of attributes. Regarding cardinality constraints, both minimum and maximum cardinalities can usually be represented, except for SHOE, RDF(S), and FLogic. In FLogic minimum cardinalities cannot be represented and maximum cardinalities can only be 1 or N (unspecified). Table 1.2 also shows whether it is possible to attach procedures to attributes or not. Only LOOM and OCML allow representing that kind of knowledge.

Concept taxonomies structure the domain concepts in a hierarchical way. The *subclass of* relationship between concepts is provided by all languages since this is the basic way to define these hierarchies. More complex knowledge such as partitions, and disjoint and exhaustive concept decompositions cannot be represented in languages like OKBC, SHOE, XOL, and RDF(S).

Sometimes the same knowledge can be represented with different modeling components. For example, disjointness in DAML+OIL and FLogic is implemented differently: in DAML+OIL special KR primitives are provided to represent disjointness, while in FLogic we must use formal axioms to represent disjointness. That is the reason why the corresponding cell in DAML+OIL contains the symbol '+' and the cell in FLogic contains the symbol 'W'.

Another example is related to partitions. In DAML+OIL partitions are defined with the primitive *daml:disjointUnionOf* ('+'). In OWL partitions must be defined in two steps ('W'): first, by expliciting that the concepts in the partition are disjoint; and second, by defining the parent concept as the union of all the concepts in the partition.

All languages allow representing binary **relations** between concepts. In many languages, attributes and relations are represented with the same primitives, although they have different ranges - datatypes and concepts respectively -. Relations of higher arity must be normally created by reification (representing them as concepts).

Relation hierarchies can be represented in the DL-based languages, Ontolingua, and OCML. In FLogic these hierarchies can be represented with formal axioms ('W'). More complex constraints, such as general integrity constraints on relations, can be only expressed by those languages that allow representing formal axioms.

Functions are very similar to relations. There are important differences between languages with respect to the arity of functions. Except for SHOE and RDF(S), binary functions can be defined (either directly or using workarounds) in all the languages. However, n-ary functions cannot be represented in ontology markup languages, but can be represented in all the classical languages except for OKBC.

Finally, we will comment on the other ontology components: instances, formal axioms, rules, procedures, etc.

With regard to **instances**, all the languages allow creating instances of the concepts and of the relations defined in an ontology. In the case of RDF(S), OIL, DAML+OIL and OWL, instances are represented in RDF.

As for **formal axioms**, most of the ontology markup languages (except SHOE and XOL) rely on a future "logic layer" that must be built on top of them, and that will provide extra logical features not provided by the languages themselves. This layered structure is shown in figure 1.5, which complements what was shown in figure 1.2: the lower part contains the XML language, which acts as the syntax of all the ontology markup languages; RDF and RDF Schema are defined on top of XML; OIL, DAML+OIL, and OWL are included in the ontology support layer, which is defined on top of RDF Schema; and the logic layer is on top of this ontology support layer.

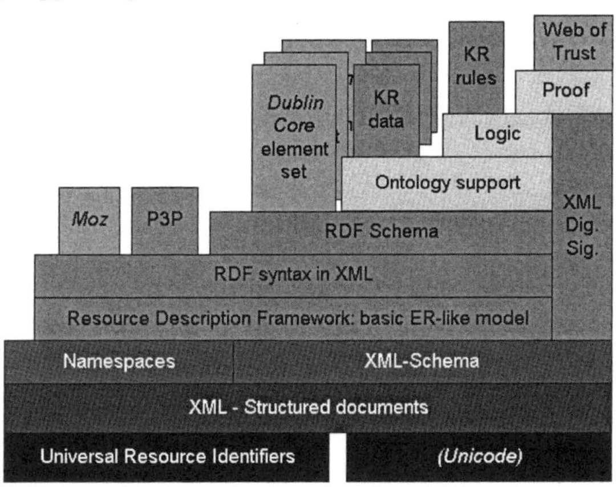

Figure 1.5. Layered structure of the Semantic Web [Berners-Lee, 1999].

Some languages include **rules** as a useful extension to perform more inferences with the language. In the cases of LOOM and OCML, the chaining mechanism of these rules (backward or forward) can be determined in the rule definition. In ontology markup languages, the logic layer will also provide support for rules, as shown in figure 1.5.

Finally, **procedures** can be created in Ontolingua, LOOM, and OCML, since these three languages are based on Lisp. Consequently, procedures in these languages must be defined in Lisp and can be executed in the KR systems associated to them[16].

1.4 Ontology Tools

To build ontologies is complex and time consuming, but it could be even more laborious if ontology developers had to implement them directly in an ontology language, without any kind of tool support. To ease this task, in the mid-1990s the first ontology building environments were created. They provided interfaces that helped users carry out some of the main activities of the ontology development process such as conceptualization, implementation, consistency checking, and documentation. In the last few years, the number of ontology tools has greatly increased and these have been diversified. [Gómez-Pérez, 2002] distinguishes the following groups:

- *Ontology development tools.* This group includes tools and integrated suites that can be used to build a new ontology from scratch. In addition to the common edition and browsing functions, these tools usually give support to ontology documentation, ontology export and import to/from different formats and ontology languages, ontology graphical edition, ontology library management, etc.
- *Ontology evaluation tools.* These are used to evaluate the content of ontologies and their related technologies. Ontology content evaluation tries to reduce problems when we need to integrate and use ontologies and ontology-based technology in other information systems.
- *Ontology merge and alignment tools.* These tools are used to solve the problem of merging and aligning different ontologies in the same domain.
- *Ontology-based annotation tools.* With these tools users can insert instances of concepts and of relations in ontologies and maintain (semi)automatically ontology-based markups in Web pages. Most of these tools have appeared recently, within the context of the Semantic Web.
- *Ontology querying tools and inference engines.* These allow querying ontologies and performing inferences with them. Normally, they are strongly related to the language used to implement ontologies.
- *Ontology learning tools.* They can derive ontologies (semi)automatically from natural language texts, as well as semi-structured sources and databases, by means of machine learning and natural language analysis techniques.

Some tool suites integrate tools from different groups, while some other isolated tools provide a limited set of functions. This section is focused only on the first group of ontology tools: those strictly used for ontology development.

1.4.1 Ontology Development Tool Evolution

Ontology development tools technology has improved enormously since the creation of the first environments. If we consider the evolution of ontology development tools since they appeared in the mid-1990s, two groups can be distinguished[17]:

---

[16] *[Levesque, 1984] defines a knowledge representation system as a server supporting two kinds of operations: telling the system additional information and asking queries. He also states that, unlike other systems, KR systems use not only explicitly told but also inferred information, in answering questions.*

- Tools whose knowledge model maps directly to an ontology language. These tools were developed as ontology editors for a specific language. This group includes the following: the Ontolingua Server [Farquhar et al., 1997], which supports ontology construction with Ontolingua and KIF; OntoSaurus [Swartout et al., 1997] with LOOM; WebOnto [Domingue, 1998] with OCML; and OilEd [Bechhofer et al., 2001a] first with OIL, then with DAML+OIL, and now with OWL.
- Integrated tool suites whose main characteristic is that they have an extensible architecture, and whose knowledge model is usually independent of an ontology language. These tools provide a core set of ontology related services and are easily extended with other modules to provide more functions. This group includes Protégé-2000 [Noy et al., 2000], WebODE [Arpírez et al., 2003], OntoEdit [Sure et al., 2002], and KAON [Maedche et al., 2003].

We are now going to present how this evolution took place and to highlight the most relevant features of all these tools.

As commented above, the main characteristic of the first group of tools is that they have a strong relationship with a specific ontology language. These tools were created to edit and browse ontologies in their corresponding languages and to import and export ontologies from/to some other ontology languages. These tools require that users have a sound knowledge of their underlying ontology language.

The **Ontolingua Server** [Farquhar et al., 1997] was the first ontology tool created. It appeared in the mid-1990s, and was built to ease the development of Ontolingua ontologies with a form-based Web interface. Initially the main application inside the Ontolingua Server was the ontology editor. Then other systems were included in the environment such as a Webster, an equation solver, an OKBC server, the ontology merge tool Chimaera, etc.

At the same time, **OntoSaurus** [Swartout et al., 1997] was implemented as a Web editor and browser for LOOM ontologies. OntoSaurus consists of two main modules: an ontology server, which uses the knowledge representation system attached to the LOOM language, and a Web browser, which allows editing and browsing LOOM ontologies with HTML forms.

In 1997, **WebOnto** [Domingue, 1998] was released. WebOnto is an ontology editor for OCML ontologies. The main difference with respect to the previous tools lay in that the ontology editor was not based on HTML forms but on Java applets, and its great advantage over the rest of ontology development tools was its strong support for collaborative ontology edition, which allowed synchronous and asynchronous discussions about the ontologies being built by groups of users.

OilEd [Bechhofer et al., 2001a] was developed in 2001 as an ontology editor for OIL ontologies. With the creation of DAML+OIL, OilEd was adapted to manage DAML+OIL ontologies and later on it was adapted to manage OWL. Users of OilEd should know how to model ontologies using a DL approach. OilEd provides consistency checking functions and automatic concept classifications by means of the FaCT inference engine [Horrocks et al., 1999], though other DL inference engines such as RACER [Haarslev and Möller, 2001] can also be used.

In recent years a new generation of ontology-engineering environments has been developed. The design rationale for these environments is much more ambitious than that of previous tools. They are built as integrated tool suites that provide technological support

[17] *In each group, a chronological order of appearance has been followed. Note that sometimes the most important bibliographic reference of a tool may have been written several years later than its first release.*

to a wide variety of activities of the ontology development process. For this purpose, they have extensible, component-based architectures where new modules can easily be added to provide more functions to the suite. Besides, the knowledge models underlying these environments are usually language independent and provide translations from and to several languages and formats.

Protégé-2000 [Noy et al., 2000] is an open source, standalone application with an extensible architecture. The core of Protégé-2000 is its ontology editor, which can be extended with plug-ins that add more functions to the environment, such as ontology language import and export (FLogic, Jess, OIL, XML, Prolog), OKBC access, constraints creation and execution (PAL), ontology merge (PROMPT), etc. Recently, a new plug-in has been created to develop OWL ontologies. However, this plug-in is not compatible with many of other existing plug-ins, since it relies heavily on a specific extension of the tool's knowledge model to deal with ontologies implemented in that language.

WebODE [Arpírez et al., 2003] is also an extensible ontology-engineering suite based on an application server, whose development started in 1999. The core of WebODE is its ontology access service, which is used by all the services and applications plugged into the server. The WebODE's Ontology Editor, which allows editing and browsing WebODE ontologies, is based on HTML forms and Java applets. The workbench integrates services for ontology language import and export (XML, RDF(S), OIL, DAML+OIL, OWL, CARIN [Levy and Rousset, 1998], FLogic, Jess, Prolog), for axiom edition with WAB (WebODE Axiom Builder), for documentation, for evaluation, for merge, and for inference. WebODE can also interoperate with Protégé-2000. The examples shown throughout this document belong to the ontology translation systems developed for WebODE, especially the translation systems for the languages RDF(S) and OWL, and for the ontology tool Protégé-2000.

OntoEdit [Sure et al., 2002] is an extensible and flexible environment based on a plug-in architecture. Its ontology editor is a standalone application that allows editing and browsing ontologies and includes functions for collaborative ontology building, inferencing, handling of domain lexicons, etc. OntoEdit exports and imports ontologies in different formats (XML, FLogic, RDF(S), and DAML+OIL), and appears in two versions: OntoEdit Free and OntoEdit Professional.

The **KAON** tool suite [Maedche et al., 2003] is an open source extensible ontology engineering environment. The core of this tool suite is the ontology API, which defines its underlying knowledge model based on an extension of RDF(S). The OI-modeller is the ontology editor of the tool suite that provides capabilities for ontology evolution, ontology mapping, ontology generation from databases, etc.

1.4.2 Comparison of Ontology Tools

Section 1.3.2 has described the formal, semi-formal and informal approaches used to compare the expressiveness of ontology languages, that can help in the task of developing ontology translation systems between languages. Clearly, these approaches can be also used to compare the knowledge models of ontology tools, to help in the provision of interoperability solutions between them and also between tools and languages and vice versa.

Table 1.3 shows the underlying KR formalism in which each tool is based, together with their underlying knowledge representation and formal axiom languages. These features determine most of the components to be used when building ontologies with them.

The table shows that the knowledge models of most of the tools are based on a combination of frames and first order logic (FOL). Only OntoSaurus and OilEd are based on description logic. The table also shows that OilEd, the Ontolingua Server, OntoSaurus and WebOnto are based on existing ontology languages, while the other tools are language-independent (except for formal axioms in OntoEdit, which are expressed in FLogic).

Table 1.3. Ontology tools' KR paradigm and underlying KR languages (updated from [Gómez-Pérez et al., 2003]).

	KAON	**OilEd**	**OntoEdit**	**Ontolingua Server**	**OntoSaurus**	**Protégé-2000**	**WebODE**	**WebOnto**
KR formalism	Frames	DL	Frames + FOL	Frames + FOL	DL	Frames + FOL	Frames + FOL	Frames + FOL
Underlying KR language	--	OWL	--	Ontolingua	LOOM	--	--	OCML
Formal axiom language	--	--	FLogic	KIF	LOOM	PAL	WAB	OCML

Table 1.4 shows the results of applying the semi-formal evaluation framework presented in section 1.3.2.2 to the ontology tools knowledge models. As we can easily infer from their relationship with existing ontology languages, the results for OilEd, the Ontolingua Server, OntoSaurus, and WebOnto are almost equivalent to those obtained for OWL DL, Ontolingua, LOOM, and OCML, respectively. The only differences that appear are mainly related to those places where a workaround was proposed in table 1.2, since some ontology tool editors restrict the components that can be represented in their underlying language.

Table 1.4. Informal comparison of ontology tools' knowledge model expressiveness (adapted from [Gómez-Pérez et al., 2003]).

	KAON	**OilEd**	**OntoEdit**	**Ontolingua Server**	**OntoSaurus**	**Protégé-2000**	**WebODE**	**WebOnto**
CONCEPTS	+	+	+	+	+	+	+	+
Metaclasses	+	-	-	+	-	+	+	-
Attributes								
Instance attributes	+	+	+	+	+	+	+	+
Class attributes	W	-	-	+	-	+	+	+
Facets								
Type constraints	+	+	+	+	+	+	+	+
Cardinality constraints	+	+	+	+	+	+	+	+
Procedural knowledge	-	-	-	-	+	-	-	+
CONCEPT TAXONOMIES								
Subclass-Of	+	+	+	+	+	+	+	+
Disjoint-Decomposition	-	+	W	+	+	W	+	+
Exhaustive-Decomposition	-	W	W	+	-	W	+	W
Partition	-	W	W	+	+	W	+	+
RELATIONS								
Binary relations	+	+	+	+	+	+	+	+
n-ary relations	W	W	W	+	+	W	+	+
Relation hierarchies	+	+	W	+	+	+	W	+
Integrity constraints	-	-	+	+	+	+	+	+
FUNCTIONS								
Binary functions	-	+	+	+	+	+	+	+
n-ary functions	-	-	+	+	+	-	-	+
OTHER COMPONENTS								
Instances	+	+	+	+	+	+	+	+
Formal Axioms	-	-	+	+	+	+	+	+
Rules	-	-	-	-	+	-	+	+
Procedures	-	-	-	+	+	-	-	+

Finally, table 1.5 summarizes the interoperability features available in the previous tools, that is, it summarizes the tools and applications where the ontologies developed with each tool can be used and how the ontologies implemented in other languages or tools can be imported. The table shows first some of the tools with which each tool can interoperate. It contains knowledge portals such as KAON-Portal and ODESeW, for KAON and WebODE respectively; ontology-based annotators such as ODEAnnotate, OntoAnnotate, and MnM; Semantic Web Services building tools, such as ODESWS; UML modeling tools, such as ArgoUML; ontology merge tools, such as Chimaera and PROMPT; etc. In some of these tools OKBC is also included because any other applications could access their ontologies by means of this protocol.

The table also shows the lists of import and export formats of each tool, providing a good overview of their interoperability choices. The lists contain ontology languages (Ontolingua, LOOM, RDF(S), DAML+OIL, OWL, etc.), general purpose languages (Prolog, Jess, etc.), and programming languages (C++, Java, etc.).

At first sight it may seem that two tools can interoperate if they share some import/export format. However, as we will describe in chapter 4, this is not necessarily true, because much knowledge can be lost during the translation process or can be translated in such a way that it is difficult to process by the target tool.

Table 1.5. Ontology tools' interoperability (adapted from [Gómez-Pérez et al., 2003]).

	KAON	**OilEd**	**OntoEdit**	**Ontolingua Server**	**OntoSaurus**	**Protégé-2000**	**WebODE**	**WebOnto**
With other tools	KAON-Portal	--	OntoAnnotate OntoMat Semantic Miner	Chimaera OKBC	OKBC	PROMPT OKBC ArgoUML	ODE-KM ODE-SeW ODE-SWS ODEAnnotate Protégé-2000	MnM
Import	KAON RDF(S)	RDF(S) OIL DAML+OIL SHIQ	OXML RDF(S) DAML+OIL FLogic	Ontolingua KIF CML IDL	LOOM PowerLOOM Stella IDL	XML RDF(S) OWL XMLS XMI	XML RDF(S) DAML+OIL OWL CARIN	OCML RDF(S)
Export	KAON RDF(S)	RDF(S) OIL DAML+OIL OWL SHIQ DIG	OXML RDF(S) DAML+OIL FLogic	Ontolingua KIF LOOM CLIPS CML Epikit Prolog IDL	LOOM PowerLOOM KIF Ontolingua Stella IDL C++	XML RDF(S) OWL XMLS FLogic CLIPS Java XMI	XML RDF(S) OIL DAML+OIL OWL CARIN FLogic Prolog Jess Java	OCML Ontolingua RDF(S)

This section has focused on comparing the expressiveness of the ontology tools' knowledge models, and on their interoperability with other tools by means of common interchange languages. There are more aspects of ontology tools that could be compared, such as their software architecture, the technology used to implement them, their ontology edition and browsing functions (including inference services attached, documentation options, logical expression editors, collaborative ontology construction, etc.), etc. However these aspects are less related to the objective of building ontology translation systems, and consequently they have not been considered in this section. Such comparisons can be found in [Gómez-Pérez, 2002] and [Gómez-Pérez et al., 2003].

1.5 The Ontology Translation Problem

As shown in the previous two sections, there is a wide variety of languages and tools for building ontologies. The ontology translation problem [Gruber, 1993a] occurs when an ontology developer decides to reuse an ontology (or part of an ontology) with a tool or language that is different from those where the ontology is available. If ontology-based system developers are forced, individually, to commit to the task of translating and incorporating the necessary ontologies to their systems, they will need great effort and much time to achieve their objectives.

According to Gruber [Gruber, 1993b], the ontology translation problem would be ameliorated if ontology developers observed the *minimal encoding bias* design criterion when building their ontologies. This criterion states that "the conceptualization should be specified at the knowledge level [Newell, 1982] without depending on a particular symbol-level encoding. The encoding bias of an axiomatization, that is, representation choices that are made purely for the convenience of notation or implementation, should be minimized".

However this design criterion is not always observed by ontology developers, because they normally use the specific features of a language or tool when building ontologies. Therefore, ontology reuse will be highly boosted as long as automatic ontology translation services among those languages and/or tools are provided.

Up to now, the work on ontology translation has mainly focused on developing translation systems for ontology tools, to import and export ontologies from and to various ontology languages. Little work has been devoted to the direct translation between ontology languages, and there are not works on the direct exchange between ontology tools without the use of common interchange languages.

1.5.1 Characterization of Ontology Translation Problems

Several classifications of ontology translation problems can be found in the literature ([Chalupsky, 2000], [Klein, 2001], [Euzenat, 2001]). It should be noticed that most of them are not specific to ontology translation per se but related to more general objectives such as semantic interoperability, or ontology merge and integration, where ontology translation may be needed at some point.

[Chalupsky, 2000] defines several levels of ontology translation problems (also known as mismatches). There are problems strictly related to the differences between the source and target formats: syntax and expressivity. Other problems are related to how an ontology has been modeled and to its ontological commitments: modeling conventions (which refers to the way in which an ontology has been modeled), model coverage and granularity (which refers to the domain coverage of the ontology), representation paradigm (which refers to the theories used for some specific parts of the domain, such as the representation of time, space, etc.), and inference system bias (which refers to how the ontology is constructed with respect to the inferences expected to be done with it).

[Klein, 2001] deals with translation problems from the ontology combination point of view. His classification is based on four levels: syntax, logical representation, semantics of primitives, and language expressivity. The first level corresponds to Chalupsky's syntax level. The other three correspond to Chalupsky's expressivity level, with slight differences between each other, which are explained in depth in [Klein, 2001]. All of these problems are tightly related to the ontology translation problem.

Finally, [Euzenat, 2001] also deals with translation problems in the context of semantic interoperability, distinguishing the following non-strict levels of language interoperability: encoding, lexical, syntactic, semantic, and semiotic[18]. He considers that the transformations can be set at these various levels, although in the approach that he presents (families of

[18] *Euzenat uses the term semiotic as a synonym of pragmatic. In linguistics, these two terms are not synonyms, since semiotics is composed of three levels: syntax, semantics and pragmatics [Morris, 1938].*

ontology languages, described in the next section) he only considers for ontology translation those that appear in the semantic level.

Figure 1.6 shows the relationships between all these layers, and with respect to the syntax, semantic and pragmatic layers defined in the area of semiotics [Morris, 1938], described in section 1.3.2.1. As we can see in the figure, the classification proposed by Euzenat is the most exhaustive one, since it considers the problems that may appear in the pragmatic layer.

[Morris, 1938]	*[Chalupsky,2000]*	*[Klein,2001]*	*[Euzenat,2001]*
Pragmatic			Semiotic
Semantic	Expressivity	Language expressivity Semantics of primitives Logical representation	Semantic
Syntax	Syntax	Syntax	Syntax Lexical Encoding

Figure 1.6. Relationships among different characterizations of ontology translation problems, and with the syntax, semantic and pragmatic layers of the theory of signs.

1.5.2 Translation Approaches and Architectures

The following three translation approaches or architectures have been distinguished in the literature (based on [Euzenat and Stuckenschmidt, 2003] and [Stuckenschmidt, 2003]):

- *Peer-to-peer translations* (aka *mapping approach*). This is the most common approach to ontology translation. Translation systems rely on ad-hoc solutions for translating between two different formats, mapping certain types of expressions in the source format to their corresponding expressions in the target format. Most of the import and export services of ontology development tools can be included in this group, such as those of the Ontolingua server, OntoSaurus, OntoEdit, OilEd, Protégé-2000, WebODE, the DAML+OIL to OWL converter[19], etc.

- *Common interchange language* (aka *pivot approach*). This approach consists in using a single pivot language to and from which all other formats are translated. To preserve semantics in the translation process, the pivot language has to be expressive enough to allow representing the knowledge that can be expressed in the source and target formats. However, if the pivot language is too expressive, it normally allows expressing the same knowledge in different ways, which makes its use difficult for achieving interoperability between any pair of source and target formats.

  An example of such a pivot language is KIF. Besides, due to the ontology language standardization process promoted by the W3C (the World Wide Web Consortium), RDF(S) and OWL can be also considered as common ontology interchange languages. Chapter 4 describes the main advantages and disadvantages of this approach, analyzing how KIF, RDF(S) and OWL have been used as common interchange languages between languages and tools. Besides, it should be noticed that the translations to and from the pivot language are created using the same kind of mappings between expressions described previously.

[19] *http://www.mindswap.org/2002/owl.html*

- *Families of ontology languages* [Euzenat and Stuckenschmidt, 2002]. This is a more formal and well-documented approach to the ontology translation problem. This approach considers having a predefined set of languages structured by a partial order relation of language coverage. The transformations to be performed between them are studied in advance and it is possible to know which are the knowledge losses between them. To perform a transformation, one of the languages in this set must be selected as the input language and another must be selected as the output language. Then several transformations are composed to transform from the source to the target format. The main drawback of this approach is that it is heavily based on description logic and that it is not clear how the approach can be used for transformations between formats not based on this KR formalism. Besides, it does not cover all the interoperability levels proposed in [Euzenat, 2001], but only translation problems related to semantic preservation.

[Euzenat and Stuckenschmidt, 2003] propose an additional architecture, based on languages composed of several layers with different expressiveness and reasoning capabilities, such as OIL and OWL. However, this approach can be considered as a specific part of the pivot one and hence it is not included in the previous list.

Figure 1.7 summarizes how these three architectures would allow performing translations among *n* formats, and shows the approximate number of ontology translation systems that would be needed in each case.

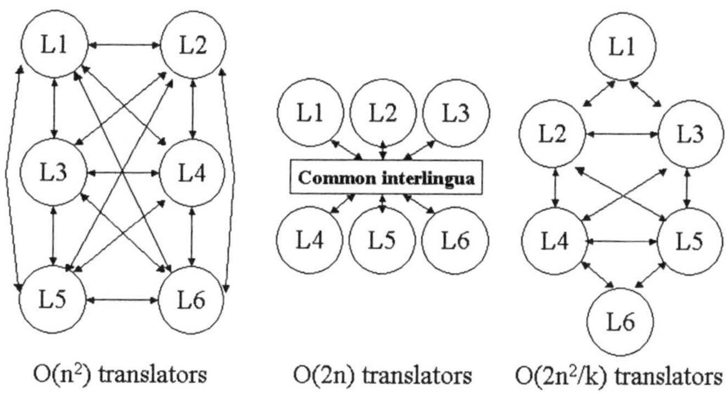

Figure 1.7. Comparison of the three architectures for ontology translation between *n* formats (adapted from [Uschold and Grüninger, 1996]).

If a unique translation system must be designed for every two party exchange, $O(n^2)$ translators would be required to achieve interoperability among *n* different KR systems. If a common interchange format is used instead, the number of translators needed is reduced to $O(2n)$. In the case of a family of ontology languages, the number of translation systems required depends on the number of levels of the structure formed by the language coverage relation. If this structure has *k* levels, with approximately *n/k* languages at each level, the number of translation systems required is $O(2n^2/k)$.

1.5.3 Technology for Building Ontology Translation Systems

Ontology translation systems are usually created using general-purpose programming languages, such as LISP or Java, and the mappings between expressions in the source and target languages are neither well-documented or explained.

There are only two specific tools that allow creating ontology translation systems, Transmorpher and OntoMorph:

- *Transmorpher*[20] [Euzenat and Tardif, 2001] is a tool that facilitates the definition and processing of complex transformations of XML documents. Among other domains this tool has been used in the context of ontologies, using a set of XSLT documents that are able to transform from one DL language to another, expressed in DLML[21]. This tool is aimed at supporting the "family of ontology languages" approach.
- *OntoMorph* [Chalupsky, 2000] is a tool that allows creating translators declaratively. Transformations between the source and the target formats are specified by means of pattern-based transformation rules and are performed in two phases: syntactic rewriting and semantic rewriting. The last one needs the ontology or part of it translated into PowerLOOM, so that this KR system can be used for certain kinds of reasoning such as discovering whether a class is subclass of another, whether a relation can be applied to a concept or not, etc. This tool can be used in the context of any of the transformation architectures presented in the previous section.

1.6 Conclusions

As shown in the sections 1.1 to 1.4, not all the ontology languages and tools are based on the same KR paradigm, nor do they represent knowledge with the same ontology components. Ontology translation is a difficult task, as it does not only consist in transforming between two syntactically different formats but also it deals with higher-level transformations to ensure semantic and pragmatic preservation in the target format, that is, preservation of the knowledge represented in the source format, and of its intended meaning. Therefore, it is important to give an adequate methodological and technological support for the creation and maintenance of ontology translation systems, so that they can be built and maintained more easily and so that they ensure higher quality translations.

Section 1.5 has shown several complementary characterizations of ontology translation problems, structured at different levels. Currently there is no consensus on the exact levels to be used for classifying these problems, although all of them cover syntax and semantic problems as the most important ones to be overcome during ontology translation.

Section 1.5 has also described three different translation approaches that have been proposed in the literature. These approaches have been usually compared to each other taking into account the number of ontology translation systems needed for performing transformations between *n* formats. In this sense, the common interchange format approach is the best option, since it reduces significantly the number of translation systems needed. However, except for the "family of ontology languages" approach, there are no deep studies about how semantics and pragmatics are preserved in these transformations, and the approaches have not been compared to each other taking into account such knowledge preservation features.

Finally, only two systems have been built specifically for developing ontology translation systems: Transmorpher and OntoMorph. They allow specifying translation decisions declaratively, what helps when developing and maintaining the translation system. However, they do not cover all the levels of translation problems that may appear in a transformation nor are they related to any method for building ontology translation systems.

The analysis of the current state of the art on ontology translation shows that there is a need for a set of integrated methods and techniques and their supporting technology, to help in the complex task of developing and maintaining ontology translation systems. Most of the

[20] *http://transmorpher.inrialpes.fr/*
[21] Description Logic Markup Language. *http://co4.inrialpes.fr/xml/dlml/*

translation systems currently available have been developed ad hoc, and the translation decisions that they implement are usually difficult to understand and hidden in the source code of the systems. Besides, it is not clear nor documented how much knowledge is lost in the transformations they perform.

In this document, we aim at providing an advance on the current state of the art on ontology translation by proposing an ontology translation model that takes into account that translation decisions must be specified declaratively and at all the different translation layers identified, and which includes a method for ontology translation system development and maintenance. The document will also explore in depth different translation approaches between two formats, with special focus on how they preserve the semantics and pragmatics of the original ontology, especially in cyclic transformation processes.

Chapter 2
Work Objectives

This chapter presents the goals of our work, together with the open research problems that we aim to solve. Besides, we detail the contributions to the current state of the art, the work hypotheses, the assumptions considered as a starting point for this work and the restrictions of the results presented.

2.1 Goals and Open Research Problems

The goal of our work is to advance the current state of the art in ontology translation by providing **a model to build ontology translation systems declaratively, taking into account the following layers of translation problems –lexical, syntax, semantic, and pragmatic–**; and by proposing **solutions that ensure semantic and pragmatic preservation** in the translation processes, especially in the case of cyclic transformations.

In order to achieve the first objective, the following (non exhaustive) list of open research problems must be solved:

- There is no consensus about the classification of ontology translation problems. Several characterizations have been proposed under different perspectives (ontology translation, ontology merge and integration, semantic interoperability, etc.), where the same problem can be classified under different groups.
- From a methodological perspective, we lack integrated methods and techniques that support the complex task of building ontology translation systems. Existing systems are usually built without considering that translation decisions can be taken at different layers. Therefore, the criteria used on the translation are not clear and the translation systems are difficult to maintain since the translation decisions are hidden inside their source code.
- From a technological perspective, there are two open problems:
  - Existing KR language comparison approaches only allow comparing KR languages, but they do not specify how to build ontology translation systems between them. Some of these approaches ([Baader, 1996] and [Borgida, 1996]) rely on the use of translation functions between two languages to compare their expressiveness.
  - There are only two systems that give technological support to the task of building ontology translation systems: OntoMorph [Chalupsky, 2000] and Transmorpher [Euzenat and Tardif, 2001]. However, they impose important limits regarding the languages to which they can be applied: the former can only be applied to Lisp-based languages and the latter can only be applied to XML-based languages.

With regard to the second objective (ensuring semantic and pragmatic preservation in translations), the following (non exhaustive) list of open research problems must be solved:

- Some ontology building methodologies consider that it may be necessary to make transformations of ontologies between different formats (Methontology [Fernández-López et al., 1999] and On-To-Knowledge [Staab et al., 2001]). Other works describe the lifecycle of ontologies once they are developed ([Gómez-Pérez and Rojas, 1999]). However, neither of these works describe in detail how knowledge is preserved when it is being translated between different formats.
- There are not detailed studies about the different approaches used so far for ontology translation and about their impact on the preservation of the semantics and pragmatics of the transformed ontologies, especially in the case of cyclic transformations.

2.2 Contributions to the State of the Art

In this document, we aim at giving solutions to the previous open research problems. Chapter 3 will describe the solutions proposed for the first objective (the creation of a layered declarative model for building and maintaining ontology translation systems) and chapter 4 will describe the solutions related to the second one (the preservation of the ontology semantics and pragmatics in translation processes).

With regard to the first objective, the document presents new advances in the state of the art in the following aspects:

- **A refinement of Euzenat's classification of ontology translation problems** ([Euzenat, 2001]), based on the theory of signs (aka semiotics). The classification proposed takes into account four different layers of translation problems: lexical, syntax, semantic, and pragmatic. It merges Euzenat's encoding and lexical layers into a single one: the lexical layer. It also considers pragmatics (the use and interpretation of the knowledge transformed) instead of semiotics (which covers, in the theory of signs, the syntax, semantic and pragmatic levels).
- **An integrated method for building ontology translation systems**, which takes into account the ontology translation layers previously identified and proposes implementing declaratively the ontology translation decisions for each layer. This method identifies the main activities and tasks to be performed, the participants of each task, and the techniques to be used in each task.
- **A language (ODEDialect) composed of three declarative languages (ODELex, ODESyntax, and ODESem),** which provide means to express and build declaratively the translation functions defined for the formal comparison approaches of KR languages and tool knowledge models. These languages improve the support provided by other tools used for building ontology translation systems as follows:
    - With regard to OntoMorph: (1) ODEDialect uses four layers to implement ontology translation decisions while OntoMorph only uses two (syntax and semantic rewriting); (2) ODEDialect does not impose the restriction of having to know an intermediate KR language (PowerLoom) to perform complex intermediate transformations; (3) ODEDialect deals with languages and tools APIs instead of dealing directly with the ontology source code (which must be in Lisp-like syntax in OntoMorph); and (4) ODEDialect uses Java instead of Lisp, the former language being more widely used for ontology technology than the latter.
    - With regard to Transmorpher: (1) ODEDialect deals with different layers of ontology translation problems separately rather than using a single XSLT file to

implement all of them; and (2) ODEDialect does not impose the restriction that the ontologies must be transformed to and from XML syntax.

The second objective deals with the preservation of the ontology semantics and pragmatics in translation processes. This document presents advances in the current state of the art in the following aspects:

- **A description of the knowledge lifecycle during translation processes**, paying special attention to cyclic transformations. As stated in the previous section, there are not detailed studies about the knowledge preservation when ontologies are translated back and forth between different formats.
- **An empirical analysis of the ontology translation approaches used for exchanging ontologies between ontology tools**. We pay special attention to how each of these approaches preserves knowledge during the translation process, by using auxiliary ontology components if necessary. It also focuses on the pragmatic preservation during the translation process, analyzing how the ontology legibility is guaranteed in the target format and how the initial ontology components are recovered in cyclic transformations. This analysis considers some ideas about the notational efficacy and conciseness of presentation of KR systems [Woods, 1983], and about the generation of auxiliary ontology components [Baader, 1996].

The layered declarative method for ontology translation described in chapter 3 gives support to cyclic transformations with semantic and pragmatic preservation.

All these contributions are backed up by a large number of experiments. These experiments show how the methodological and technological solutions proposed have been applied to real-world problems, tackled in the context of the following R&D projects: the EU funded MKBEEM[22] and Esperonto[23] projects, and the Spanish CICYT funded ContentWeb project (TIC-2001-2745).

2.3 Work Assumptions, Hypothesis, and Restrictions

The work described in this document is based on the set of **assumptions** listed below. These assumptions help explain the decisions taken for the development of the methodological and technological solutions and the relevance of the contributions presented. Assumptions A1 to A3 are related to our first objective, whilst the assumption A4 deals with the second one.

A1. The boundaries between different layers of ontology translation problems are not strict, that is, some translation problems may be related to several layers and the decisions taken at one layer may influence the decisions taken at the others.

A2. Ontology translation systems are complex software systems: they are difficult to create and maintain, and the translation decisions taken are normally difficult to understand. They are easier to create, maintain, and reuse if they are implemented taking into account different layers of ontology translation problem and using a declarative approach.

A3. An ontology translation system is a software system. Therefore, any software engineering methodology can be applied to its construction. However, specific activities and tasks can be inserted in the software engineering methodology to help build these systems more efficiently and with higher quality.

---

[22] IST-1999-10589. *http://www.mkbeem.com/*

[23] IST-2001-34373. *http://www.esperonto.net/*

A4. An ontology translation system does not necessarily have to preserve the semantics and the pragmatics of the ontology that it transforms. These preservation properties, which are normally desirable features, depend on the foreseen application of the ontologies transformed with such a system.

Once the assumptions have been identified and presented, the set of **hypothesis** of our work are described. This set of hypothesis covers the main features of the proposed solutions:

H1. The layered declarative ontology translation model combines existing translation proposals and techniques (used for describing languages and tools, for comparing them, for deciding the feasibility of the construction of an ontology translation system, etc.), and eases the task of expressing translation decisions between two formats.

H2. The method proposed as part of the ontology translation model gives an integrated support to the four ontology translation layers identified. The method proposes using specific techniques to solve the problems of each layer and using declarative languages to implement the transformations at each layer.

H3. The method proposed distinguishes several user roles in charge of different tasks. Of these roles the most important one is the knowledge engineer, who is in charge of analyzing, designing and implementing the transformations between the source and target formats. This person must have a deep knowledge of the source and target formats' knowledge models, and of their ontology management APIs.

H4. The proposed method and technology are independent of the ontology translation architecture where they are used. Hence, they can be applied to construct translation systems in pivot approaches, peer-to-peer translations, and in the "family of ontology languages" approach.

H5. The proposed method and technology can be applied to construct ontology translation systems independently of the requirements imposed with regard to semantic and pragmatic preservation.

Finally, the following set of **restrictions** defines the limits of our contributions and allows determining future research objectives. Most of these restrictions are related to the technological aspects of the contribution (R1 to R6), while R7 deals with the study about semantic and pragmatic preservation and R8, R9, and R10 are related to the experimentation.

R1. The layers and the method described in this document are only proposed for the task of ontology translation. They do not aim at solving the translation problem of other types of knowledge, such as knowledge about planning, knowledge about machine learning, etc.

R2. The proposed method and technology do not consider the optimization of the translation process of the system generated, neither in terms of the space required during translation nor in terms of the time needed to complete the translation.

R3. The ontology translation systems generated from ODEDialect specifications take as an input an ontology in the source format and they output the ontology in the target format, according to the translation decisions implemented.

R4. The ODEDialect language cannot be applied to create ontology translation systems to and from languages or tools that do not provide an ontology management API in Java, unless such an API is generated prior to the development of the ontology translation system.

R5. Ontology translation systems developed with the ODEDialect language do not make incremental translations, nor are they connected to ontology version control management methods or tools.

R6. The three declarative languages that compose ODEDialect (ODELex, ODESyntax, and ODESem) are not expressive enough to represent every possible type of transformation that may appear in any transformation. They only cover the most common types of transformations identified at each layer. If a more complex transformation must be performed, user-defined functions must be used.

R7. The description of semantic and pragmatic preservation during translation processes is restricted to the "representational aspects" of the origin and target formats [Baader, 1996]. It does not encompass other aspects such as the reasoning tractability of the knowledge generated in the target format.

R8. The proposed model has been derived from the experimentation on building WebODE import and export services from and to different types of ontology and other general-purpose languages, such as DAML+OIL, OIL, XCARIN, FLogic, Java, and XML.

R9. Once created, the evaluation of the proposed ontology translation model is restricted to the ontology markup languages RDF(S) and OWL, and to the ontology tools Protégé-2000 and WebODE. They have been selected because RDF(S) and OWL are the current W3C recommendations for the Semantic Web, Protégé-2000 is the most widely-used ontology tool, and WebODE has been developed inside the Ontological Engineering Group to which the author belongs.

R10. The results shown in the experimentation chapter are based on the use of the following versions of the ontology tools and languages: Protégé-2000 version 2.0, WebODE version 2.0, and RDF(S) and OWL recommendations of February 2004.

Chapter 3
A Layered Declarative Ontology Translation Model

This chapter presents a model for ontology translation, based on the experience gathered in the construction of ontology translation systems between languages and/or tools. This model is characterized by two main features: on the one hand, translation decisions are defined at four different layers: lexical, syntax, semantic, and pragmatic; on the other hand, translation decisions are mainly implemented in a declarative fashion. The main assumption behind this proposal is that both aspects make ontology translation systems easier to build, maintain, and reuse. As part of this model, we propose a method for guiding during the process of developing an ontology translation system between two ontology languages and/or tools. This method consists of four activities (feasibility study, analysis of source and target formats, design of the translation system, and implementation of the translation system), which are in their turn divided into several tasks. For each task, we specify the objectives, inputs and outputs, plus a set of proposed techniques that can be used to perform the task and the main agent responsible of the task.

3.1 Introduction

This section describes a model for developing ontology translation systems between two formats, which can be either ontology languages or ontology tools. As expressed by the chapter title, there are two parameters that fully characterize this model:

- The model is ***layered***, which means that translation decisions are structured in different levels [Corcho, 2002]: lexical, syntactic, semantic, and pragmatic. These layers are related to different categories of ontology translation problems. We assume that it is more simple to create and maintain ontology translation systems where translation decisions are clearly defined in different layers because they are easier to understand, and because the automatization of the ontology translation process is also easier. Besides, the problems to be solved in each layer are different (it is not the same to transform a concept identifier from a format into another –e.g. by replacing its blank spaces with underscores– than to transform a set of logical restrictions into a disjoint decomposition of a concept). Therefore we will require using different translation techniques for each layer.
- The model is mainly ***declarative***, and this basically means that most of the translation decisions are not "hidden" inside the source code of the ontology translation system. As we will describe further in this chapter, we will use different types of tables and diagrams to formalize the translation decisions to be made at each layer, and

declarative languages to implement them (ODELex, ODESyntax, and ODESem). For instance, in the semantic layer, for each type of ontology component of the source format (e.g., concepts, relations, etc.), we will express declaratively the transformations to be performed to get the same knowledge in the target format. We will use only general-purpose programming languages (Java) for expressing complex transformations that cannot be defined declaratively.

Sections 3.2 and 3.3 describe in detail these dimensions and show examples of how transformations are expressed at each layer. It is important to remark that this model does not aim to solve the ontology translation problem per se, since its objective is not to create a generic ontology translation system for every pair of source and target formats used for representing ontologies. Instead, its aim is to improve the state-of-the-art of ontology translation by providing a structured and declarative form of expressing transformations between different formats.

Finally, section 3.4 describes in depth the ontology translation method proposed in this model. The method recommends accomplishing four main activities, which are in its turn divided into tasks. For each of these tasks, we describe the objectives, the inputs and outputs, the recommended techniques and the main participants.

3.2 Ontology Translation Layers

As we commented above, our model proposes structuring translation decisions in four different layers: lexical, syntax, semantic, and pragmatic. Our selection of layers is based on the classifications of ontology translation mismatches and interoperability levels for semantic integration shown in section 1.5, especially on Euzenat's one [Euzenat, 2001]. We will now describe the types of translation problems that can be usually found in each of these layers and we will show some examples of common transformations performed in each of them.

3.2.1 Lexical Layer

The lexical layer deals with the "ability to segment the representation in characters and words (or symbols)" [Euzenat, 2001]. Different languages and tools normally use different character sets and grammars for generating their terminal symbols (ontology component identifiers, natural language descriptions of ontology components, and attribute values). This translation layer deals with the problems that may arise in these symbol transformations.

Therefore, in this layer we deal with the following types of transformations:

- **Transformations of ontology component identifiers**. For instance, the source and target formats use different sets of characters for creating identifiers, the source and target format use different naming conventions for their component identifiers, or their components have different scopes, and hence some component identifiers cannot overlap with the identifiers of other components.
- **Transformations of pieces of text used for natural language documentation purposes**. For instance, specific characters in the natural language documentation of a component must be escaped since the target format does not allow them as part of the documentation.
- **Transformations of values**. For instance, numbers must be represented as character strings in the target format, or dates must be transformed according to the date formulation rules of the target format.

From a lexical point of view, among the most representative ontology languages and tools we can distinguish three **groups of formats**:

- *ASCII-based formats*. Among these formats we can cite the following classical languages: KIF, Ontolingua, CycL, LOOM, OCML, and FLogic. Also in this group we can include the ontology tools related to some of these languages (the Ontolingua Server, OntoSaurus, and WebOnto). These languages are based on ASCII encodings, and hence the range of characters allowed for creating ontology component identifier, and for representing natural language texts and values is restricted to most of the characters allowed in this encoding.
- *UNICODE-based formats*. Among these formats we can cite the following ontology tools: OntoEdit, Protégé-2000, and WebODE. These formats are based on the UNICODE encoding, which is an extension of the ASCII encoding and thus allows using more varied characters (including Asian and Arabic characters, more punctuation signs, etc.).
- *UNICODE&XML-based formats*. Among these formats we can refer to the ontology markup languages: SHOE, XOL, RDF, RDFS, OIL, DAML+OIL, and OWL, and some of the tools that are related to them, such as KAON and OilEd. These formats are characterized not only for being UNICODE compliant, as the previous ones, but also for restricting the use of some characters and groups of characters in the component identifiers and in the natural language documentation and values, such as the use of tag-style pieces of text (e.g., *<example>*) inside documentation tags. An important restriction is the compulsory use of qualified names (*QNames*) as identifiers of ontology concepts and properties, since they are used to construct tags when dealing with instances.

The easiest lexical transformations are usually those to be done from the first and third group of formats to the second one, which is the most unrestricted one. In other cases, the specific features of each format do not allow us to generalize the types of transformations to be done, which mainly consist in replacing non-allowed characters with others that are allowed, or in replacing identifiers that are reserved keywords in a format with other identifiers that are not. Obviously, there are also differences among the languages and tools inside each group, although the transformations needed in those cases are minimal.

Special attention deserves the problem related to the scope of the ontology component identifiers in the source and target formats, and to the restrictions related to overlapping identifiers. These problems appear when, in the source format, a component is defined inside the scope of another and thus its identifier is local to the latter, while the correspondent component has a global scope in the target format. As a consequence, there could be clashes of identifiers if two different components have the same identifier in the source format.

Table 3.1 shows some examples of how some ontology component identifiers can be transformed from WebODE to Ontolingua, RDF(S), OWL and Protégé-2000, taking into account the rules for generating identifiers in each format and the constraints about the scope and possible overlap of some ontology component identifiers.

As expressed above, inside this layer we also deal with the different naming conventions that exist in different formats[24]. For instance, in Lisp-based languages and tools such as

[24] *These types of problems may be also related to the pragmatic layer, as we will describe later in this section. We will also see that the limits of each translation layer are not strict; hence we can find transformation problems that are in the middle of several layers.*

Ontolingua, LOOM, OCML, and their corresponding ontology tools, compound names are usually joined together using hyphens: e.g. `Travel-Agency`. In tools like OntoEdit, Protégé and WebODE, words are separated with blank spaces: e.g. `Travel Agency`. In ontology markup languages, the convention used for class identifiers is to write all the words together, with no blank spaces nor hyphens, and with the first capital letter for each word: e.g. `TravelAgency`.

Table 3.1. Examples of transformations at the lexical layer.

WebODE identifier	Target	Result	Reasons for transformation
`Business Trip`	Ontolingua	`Business-Trip`	Blank spaces in identifiers are not allowed in Ontolingua
`1StarHotel`	RDF(S)	`OneStarHotel`	Identifiers cannot start with a digit in RDF(S). They do not form valid QNames
Concepts `Name` and `name`	Ontolingua	classes `Name` and `Name_1`	Ontolingua is not case sensitive
Concept `Room` attribute `fare` Concept `Flight` attribute `fare`	OWL	classes `Room`, `Flight` datatypeProperty `roomFare` datatypeProperty `flightFare`	WebODE attributes are local to concepts. OWL datatype properties are not defined in the scope of OWL classes, but globally
Concept `Name` attribute `Name`	Protégé-2000	class `Name`; slot `name`	The identifiers of classes and slots cannot overlap in Protégé-2000

3.2.2 Syntactic Layer

This layer deals with the "ability to structure the representation in structured sentences, formulas or assertions" [Euzenat, 2001]. Ontology components in each language or tool are defined with different grammars. Hence, the syntactic layer deals with the problems related to how the symbols are structured in the source and target formats, taking into account the derivation rules for ontology components in each of them.

In this layer the following types of transformations are included:

- **Transformations of ontology component definitions** according to the grammars of the source and target formats. For instance, the grammar to define a concept in Ontolingua is different than that in OCML.
- **Transformations of datatypes**. For instance, the datatype *date* in WebODE must be transformed to the datatype *&xsd;date* in OWL.

Figure 3.1 shows an example of how a WebODE concept definition (expressed in XML) is transformed into Ontolingua and OWL. In this example both types of translation problems are dealt with.

Among the most representative ontology languages and tools we can distinguish the following (overlapping) groups of formats:

- *Lisp-based formats*. In section 1.3 we showed that the syntax of several classical ontology languages are based on the Lisp language, namely KIF and Ontolingua, LOOM, and OCML, together with their corresponding ontology tools (the Ontolingua Server, OntoSaurus, and WebOnto, respectively). The Lisp language was widely used for building knowledge representation systems especially during the 1970s, the 1980s and the 1990s.

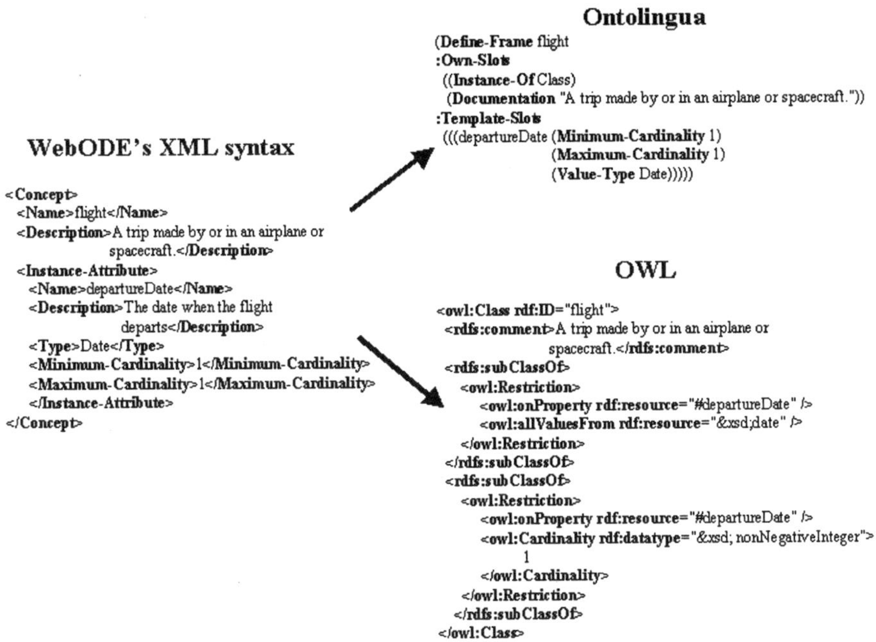

Figure 3.1. Examples of transformations at the syntactic layer.

- *XML-based formats*. As shown also in section 1.3, ontology markup languages are characterized by being represented in XML syntax. Among then we can cite: SHOE, XOL, RDF, RDFS, OIL, DAML+OIL, and OWL. In addition, ontology tools such as OntoEdit, Protégé-2000, and WebODE also provide ad hoc XML backends to implement their ontologies.
- *Ad hoc text formats*. There are other ontology languages that do not provide any of the previous syntaxes but their own ad hoc formats. These languages are F-Logic, the ASCII syntax of OIL, and the Notation-3 (N3) syntax used to represent ontologies in RDF, RDFS, and OWL. Except for F-Logic, these syntaxes are alternative and mainly intended for human-consumption.
- *Ontology management APIs*. Finally, several ontology languages and tools provide ontology management APIs. These APIs are included here because they can be considered as another form of syntax: the expressions used to access, create, and modify ontology components in the programming language in which these APIs are available have to be created according to the specification provided by the API. Among the languages with an ontology management API we have: all the ontology markup languages, where ontologies can be created using available XML Java APIs such as DOM, SAX, etc.; and, more specifically, RDF, RDFS, DAML+OIL, and OWL, for which there are specific APIs that resemble the knowledge models of the ontology languages, such as Jena, the OWL API, etc. Among the tools we have: KAON, OntoEdit, Protégé-2000, and WebODE.

There are other aspects to be considered in this layer, such as the fact that some ontology languages and tools allow defining the same component with different syntaxes. For example, Ontolingua provides at least four different ways to define concepts: using KIF, using the Frame Ontology or using the OKBC-Ontology exclusively, or embedding KIF expressions inside definitions that use the Frame Ontology [Corcho and Gómez-Pérez,

1999]. This variety adds complexity both for the generation of such a format (we must decide what kind of expression to use[25]) and for its processing (we have to take into account all the possible syntactic variants for the same piece of knowledge).

Inside this layer we must also take into account how the different formats represent datatypes. Two groups can be distinguished:

- *Formats with their own internal datatypes*. Among these formats we can refer to all the ontology languages described in section 1.3 except RDF, RDFS, and OWL, and all the ontology tools described in section 1.4.
- *Formats with XML Schema datatypes*. These datatypes have been defined with the aim of providing datatype standardization in Web contexts (e.g., in Web services). They can be used in the ontology languages RDF, RDFS, and OWL, and in the ontology tool WebODE, which allows using both types of datatypes (internal and XML Schema ones).

Therefore, with regard to datatypes, the problems to be solved will mainly consist in finding the relationships between the internal datatypes of the source and target formats (not all the formats have the same group of datatypes) or finding relationships between the internal datatypes of a format and the XML Schema datatypes, and vice versa.

3.2.3 Semantic Layer

This layer deals with the "ability to construct the propositional meaning of the representation" [Euzenat, 2001]. Different ontology languages and tools can be based on different KR paradigms (frames, semantic networks, first order logic, conceptual graphs, etc.) or on combinations of them, as described in section 1.3. These KR paradigms do not always allow expressing the same type of knowledge, and sometimes the languages and tools based on these KR paradigms allow expressing the same knowledge in different ways.

Therefore, in this layer we deal not only with simple transformations (e.g., WebODE concepts are transformed into Ontolingua and OWL classes), but also with complex transformations of expressions that are usually related to the fact that the source and target formats are based on different KR paradigms (e.g., WebODE disjoint decompositions are transformed into subclass-of relationships and PAL[26] constraints in Protégé-2000, WebODE instance attributes attached to a class are transformed into datatype properties in OWL and unnamed property restrictions for the class).

As an example, figure 3.2 shows how to represent a concept partition in different ontology languages and tools. In WebODE and LOOM there are specific built-in primitives for representing partitions. In OWL the partition must be represented by defining the *rdfs:subClassOf* relationship between each class in the partition and the parent class, by stating that every possible pair of classes in the decomposition are disjoint, and by defining the parent class as the union of all the classes in the partition. In Protégé-2000 the partition is represented like in OWL, with *subclass-of* relationships between all the classes in the partition and the parent class, with several PAL constraints that represent disjointness between all the classes in the partition, and with the statement that the parent class is abstract (that is, that it cannot have direct instances).

Most of the work on ontology translation done so far has been devoted to solving semantic transformation problems. For example, the formal, semi-formal, and informal methods for comparing ontology languages and ontology tools' knowledge models, which were

---

[25] *As with naming conventions, this decision will be also related to the pragmatic translation layer.*

[26] *Protégé Axiom Language*

described in chapter 1, aim at helping to decide whether two formats have the same expressiveness or not, so that knowledge can be preserved in the transformation. And some of these approaches can be also used to decide whether the reasoning mechanisms present in both formats will allow inferring the same knowledge in the target format.

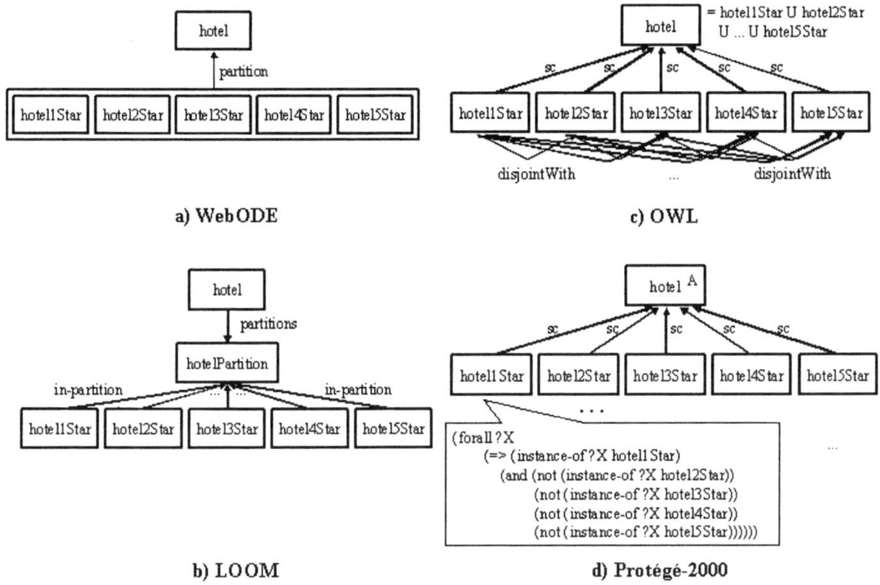

Figure 3.2. Examples of transformations at the semantic layer.

Basically, these studies permit analyzing the expressiveness (and in some cases the reasoning mechanisms) of the source and target formats so that we can know which types of components can be translated directly from a format to another, which types of components can be expressed using other types of components from the target format, which cannot be expressed in the target format, and which can be expressed in the target format, even though they may lose part of the knowledge represented in the source format.

Therefore, the catalogue of problems that can be found in this layer is mainly related to the different KR formalisms in which the source and target formats are based. This does not mean that translating between two formats based on the same KR formalism is straightforward, since there might be differences in the types of ontology components that can be represented in each of them. This is specially important in the case of DL languages, because many different combinations of primitives can be used in each language, and hence many possibilities exist in the transformations between them, as shown in [Euzenat, 2002]. However, the most interesting results are obtained when the source and target KR formalisms are different.

We will present the most relevant problems that usually appear in the transformations between the following KR formalisms: frames combined with first order logic and description logics. With regard to the description logic formalism, we will consider in the following sections that we are using a SHOIN(d+) language (the language to which OWL DL is equivalent), as it is one of the most expressive DL languages for which there are decidable reasoners.

3.2.3.1 Semantic Transformations of Combinations of Frames and First Order Logic into Description Logic

This section deals with the types of transformation problems that usually appear at the semantic layer if the source format is a language or tool based on a combination of frames and first order logic and when the target format is a language or tool based on description logic. We do not go into more detail on the specific problems that appear between specific formats of each KR paradigm. Besides, this list must not be considered exhaustive, since there are many other problems that appear at the semantic layer when transforming between formats based on both formalisms. Instead we have tried to show the most relevant ones:

- Metaclasses can be usually expressed in frame-based formats. However they cannot be expressed in description logic because of the reasoning problems they provoke. Consequently, this knowledge is normally lost in the translation.
- In the frame KR paradigm, class definitions are normally partial (that is, classes are primitive –using the DL vocabulary–, because their definition only expresses necessary conditions for instances that belong to the class). There are only two exceptions in frames where the definition of a class is not partial but complete: (1) in some languages, such as Ontolingua and OCML, it is possible to define the necessary and sufficient conditions that instances must comply with to belong to the class (with the *:iff-def* keyword); (2) and in some languages formal axioms can be also defined stating the sufficient conditions that instances must comply with to belong to the class (the necessary conditions are already provided in the class definition). The problem in this case is whether to translate a class definition of a frame-based language to a partial or complete definition in a DL language.
- Class partitions and disjoint and exhaustive class decompositions can be defined in many frame-based languages. However, most of the DL languages do not provide these primitives for building class taxonomies but only the *subclass-of* relationship. Therefore, these decompositions and partitions must be transformed using the *subclass-of* relationships. However, this knowledge is not necessarily lost, because the disjointness between classes can be expressed by stating that the class `A` is a subclass of the class `not B`. Finally, exhaustiveness in class taxonomies can be expressed in DL with complete definitions using the union of all the classes in the decomposition or partition, that is, stating that $A = C1 \cup C2 \cup \ldots \cup Cn$.
- Own slots are used to specify properties of the classes themselves in the frame-based paradigm. These slots cannot be usually expressed in DL. Consequently, this knowledge is normally lost in the transformation.
- Some frame-based systems define slots as second-class citizens of the ontology, that is, they are defined inside the scope of other ontology components (e.g., classes). On the contrary, in DL roles are always global to ontologies. To transform frame-based slots into DL roles, the roles must be defined globally and must be "attached" to classes with universal property restrictions; and their cardinality must be expressed with cardinality restrictions. Several situations may arise from these scope differences:
  - If the slot is defined in the scope of several classes, then its domain can be interpreted as the union of all those classes.
  - If the slot has several ranges, then the slot range is (usually) considered as the union of the classes in frame-based systems, while in DL it is considered as the intersection of the classes.
- Not all the axioms that can be created in FOL can be expressed in DL.

3.2.3.2 Semantic Transformations of Description Logic into Combinations of Frames and First Order Logic

Unlike in the previous case, most of the problems that can appear in the transformations in this direction (of a description logic format into a format based on a combination of frames and first order logic) can be solved by the use of FOL axioms. The most typical problems to be dealt with are:

- DL formats usually allow representing class conjunctions (intersection of classes) and class disjunctions (union of classes) as part of other class expressions, as shown in section 1.3. However, the frame-based KR paradigm cannot express class disjunctions. To transform such expressions from DL, FOL axioms must be created to express the disjunction of a set of classes. For instance, the expression `ManOrWoman`, which is defined as the union of the classes `Man` and `Woman` (`ManOrWoman = Man ∪ Woman`) is transformed into the class `ManOrWoman`, and a FOL axiom is created stating that it is the union of both: `∀x (ManOrWoman(x) ↔ Man(x) ∨ Woman(x))`
- DL permits using complex expressions inside class and role definitions that do not have identifiers, whereas in frame-based formats all the ontology components must have an identifier. Therefore, these complex anonymous expressions must be transformed into ontology components with special identifiers (anonymous classes or relations) together with FOL axioms that define them if necessary. For instance, the class *Agent* can be defined as a subclass of the union of the classes `Animal` or `Plant` (`Agent ⊆ Animal ∪ Plant`). To transform this expression into a frame-based format, the classes `Agent`, `Animal`, and `Plant` must be created plus the "anonymous" class `AnimalOrPlant` and the FOL axiom `∀x (AnimalOrPlant(x) ↔ Animal(x) ∨ Plant(x))`. Consequently, a new identifier has been created together with the FOL axiom that defines it.
- Defined (necessary and sufficient) class definitions in DL must be transformed into partial definitions in frames, plus FOL axioms to state the equivalences expressed in the definition. For instance, the class definition `Flight = Travel ∩ ∀usesTransportMean.Plane`, which states that a flight is a kind of travel that uses a plane as a transport mean, must be transformed to a frame-based format as the class `Flight`, which is subclass of the class `Travel`, and with a slot `usesTransportMean` whose range is `Plane`. Besides, the following FOL axiom must be created to state the sufficient conditions of the class:

  `∀x(Travel(x) ∧ ∀y(usesTransportMean(x,y) → Plane(y)) → Flight(x))`
- DL formats usually allow representing cycles in class taxonomies, while frame-based formats do not usually allow them. To perform such transformations, FOL axioms must be created, if they are allowed in the target format. However, from a frame-based perspective this is normally considered as a knowledge representation error.
- The DL expressions that state that a class is subclass of the complement of another class or expression (`C ⊆ ¬D`) are transformed to disjointness relationships between the classes involved in the expression.
- Universal property restrictions of classes are transformed into range restrictions of the slots in the corresponding class. Existential property restrictions of classes are transformed to minimum cardinality restrictions of the slots in the corresponding class.
- If the range of a role is not specified in a property restriction, the range of the corresponding slot must be set to the most general class in the ontology in the frame-based format.

3.2.4 Pragmatic Layer

This layer deals with the “ability to construct the pragmatic meaning of the representation (or its meaning in context)”. Therefore, in this layer we deal with the transformations to be made in the ontology resulting from the lexical, syntactic, and semantic transformations so that both human users and ontology-based applications will notice as less differences as possible with respect to the ontology in the original format, either in one-direction transformations or in cyclic transformations.

Therefore, transformations in this layer will require the following: adding special labels to ontology components so as to preserve their original identifier in the source format; transforming sets of expressions into more legible syntactic constructs in the target format; “hiding” completely or partially some ontology components not defined in the source ontology but that have been created as part of the transformations (such as the anonymous classes commented previously); etc.

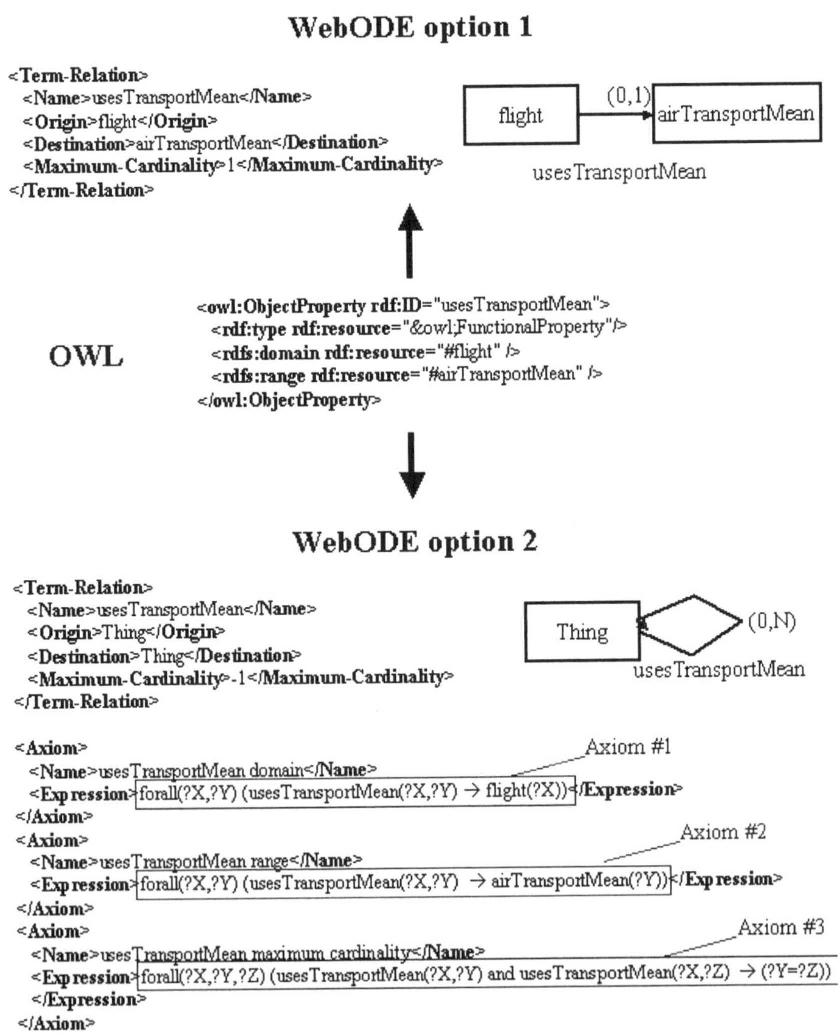

Figure 3.3. Examples of transformations at the pragmatic layer.

Figure 3.3 shows two transformations of the OWL functional object property `usesTransportMean` to WebODE. The object property domain is the class `flight` and its range is the class `airTransportMean`. The figure shows two of the possible semantically equivalent sets of expressions that can be obtained when transforming that definition. In the first one, the object property is transformed into the ad-hoc relation `usesTransportMean` that holds between the concepts `flight` and `airTransportMean`, with its maximum cardinality set to one. In the second one, the object property is transformed into the ad-hoc relation `usesTransportMean` whose domain and range is the concept `Thing` (the root of the ontology concept taxonomy), with no restrictions on its cardinality, plus three formal axioms expressed in first order logic: the first one stating that the relation domain is `flight`, the second one that its range is `airTransportMean`, and the third one imposing the maximum cardinality constraint[27].

From a human user's point of view, the first WebODE definition is more legible: at one glance the user can see that the relation `usesTransportMean` is defined between the concepts `flight` and `airTransportMean`, and that its maximum cardinality is one. In the second case, the user must find and interpret the four components (the ad-hoc relation definition and the three formal axioms) to reach the same conclusion.

A similar conclusion can be obtained from an application point of view. Let us suppose that we want to populate the ontology with an annotation tool. The behavior of the annotation tool is different for both definitions. With the first definition, the annotation tool will easily "understand" that its user interface cannot give users the possibility of adding more than one instance of the relation, and that the drop-down lists used for selecting the domain and range of a relation instance will only show direct or indirect instances of the concepts `flight` and `airTransportMean`, respectively. With the second definition, the annotation tool will allow creating more than one relation instance from the same instance and will display all the ontology instances in the drop-down lists, instead of just presenting instances of `flight` and `airTransportMean` respectively. After that, the annotation tool will have to run the consistency checker to detect inconsistencies in the ontology.

We will present the most relevant pragmatic problems that usually appear in the transformations of frames combined with first order logic into description logic. As in the previous section, we will consider that we are using a SHOIN(d+) language.

3.2.4.1 Pragmatic Transformations of Combinations of Frames and First Order Logic into Description Logic

This section describes some of the most typical transformations that must be performed at the pragmatic level when translating ontologies of a format based on a combination of frames and first order logic into another format based on description logic. As it occurred with the semantic transformations, the list of transformations is not exhaustive but indicative of the main problems that may appear in such scenario.

As expressed in section 3.2.3.2, class definitions in the frames KR formalism are always primitive (that is, they only express necessary conditions but not sufficient conditions for an instance to belong to that class). To express sufficient conditions first order logic axioms must be represented. Consequently, class definitions should be transformed into primitive class definitions in DL-based formats. The use of these types of definitions in DL-based formats may have a negative influence when reasoning with the transformed ontologies in the target format, especially in the case of instance classification. Consequently, in some

---

[27] *We must note that this second option may be obtained because expressions in OWL ontologies may appear in any order in an OWL file, and hence may be processed independently.*

cases it may be interesting to create complete definitions from the partial definitions expressed in frames, since in most of the frame-based systems this distinction is not made.

In DL, the specification of the domain and range of properties is not usually considered for reasoning, since property definitions are normally taken as atomic definitions. However, in frame-based systems, this type of information is usually provided and, although it is not necessary to transform it into DL, it could be interesting to do so, for legibility reasons, if the target format allows representing it.

As in many other target formats, independently of the KR formalism upon which they are based, DL-based formats usually provide many different ways to express the same piece of knowledge. In the pragmatic level, we must decide which of the different but semantically equivalent forms must be created from an expression in the source format. For instance, the disjointness relationship between two classes can be expressed in DL (if possible) in the following three forms: a) with a *disjointWith* primitive, b) stating that the intersection of the two classes is a subclass of the predefined class *bottom*, and c) stating that one of the classes is a subclass of the complement of the another.

3.2.4.2 Pragmatic Transformations of Description Logic into Combinations of Frames and First Order Logic

As in the previous section, here we collect and describe some common transformations that have to be performed at the pragmatic level when transforming a DL-based format into a format based on a combination of frames and first order logic. Most of these transformations are related to the avoidance of using first order logic axioms when they can be rewritten using other modeling components available in the frame-based format.

Anonymous class disjunction expressions in DL are normally transformed into anonymous classes in frame-based systems. These anonymous classes are usually defined with first order logic axioms. In order to improve the legibility of the resulting ontology after a transformation process, these anonymous classes should be easy to identify. For example, special identifiers may be used to show that the classes do not belong to the domain, or the classes may be hidden to users (this last option is normally possible only with some ontology tools, such as Protégé-2000 form personalization or WebODE views, but it is not possible with ontology languages).

DL defined classes should be transformed into classes in frame-based partial class definitions, which express necessary conditions, plus first order logic axioms, which express sufficient conditions. With this type of transformation, the semantics of the transformed expression is preserved but the legibility is lower, since many formal axioms will appear in the ontology to express this sufficient conditions. As commented in the previous section, it may not be so important to express the defined classes and it could just suffice with the partial class definitions commonly found in frame-based systems.

If a class is defined as the union of a set of classes (`A = C1 ∪ C2 ∪ ... ∪ Cn`), and these classes are defined as subclasses of that class, then the expression that would be normally obtained when transforming into a frame-based system would be: the class `A`, the classes `C1` to `Cn`, a first order logic axiom expressing that the class A is the union of all those classes, and many subclass of relationships between the classes `Ci` and the class `A`. In many frame-based systems, all this information can be expressed more compactly as an exhaustive decomposition of the class `A`. Similarly, if all the classes in the set are disjoint to each other, then the information would be expressed as a partition.

In DL all the subclass of relationships are not necessarily expressed in ontologies, since this kind of information can be extracted by their automatic classifiers. From a pragmatic point of view, in the transformation into frame-based systems it could be interesting to run the automatic classifier first in order to obtain all the *subclass-of* relationships that can be inferred from the ontology definitions, and translate also these inferred *subclass-of* relationships.

3.2.5 Relationships among Ontology Translation Layers

Figure 3.4 shows an example of a transformation of WebODE into OWL DL. In this example, we have to transform two ad hoc relations with the same name (`usesTransportMean`) and with different domains and ranges (a `flight` uses an `airTransportMean` and a `cityBus` uses a `bus`). In OWL DL the scope of an object property is global to the ontology. Therefore we cannot define two different object properties with the same name. In the example we show that translation decisions have to be taken at all layers. We also show the complexity of the translation task, because a decision taken at one layer can affect the decisions taken at the others.

Option 1 is mainly driven by semantics: in order to preserve semantics in the transformation, two different object properties are defined. Option 2 is driven by pragmatics: only one object property is defined from both ad hoc relations since we assume that they refer to the same meaning, but some knowledge is lost in the transformation (the exact information about the domain and range of the object property). Finally, option 3 is also driven by pragmatics, with more care on the semantics: again, only one object property is defined and its domain and range are more restricted than in option 2. However we still lose the exact correspondence between each domain and each range.

To sum up, in this section we have identified a catalogue of transformation problems that can appear at different layers. These problems are usually solved with different approaches and purposes. However the differences between the four translation layers described should not be considered strict. In fact, we have already showed in section 1.5 that there is no consensus about the levels where interoperability problems can appear, and we have also shown, especially when dealing with pragmatics, that translation decisions made at one layer usually affect the decisions made in the others.

3.3 Declarative Specification of Translation Decisions

As described in the previous section translation decisions can be structured in four layers: lexical, syntactic, semantic, and pragmatic. Now we present how these translation decisions can be specified declaratively, what avoids hiding translation decisions inside the source code of ontology translation systems, hence easing the creation and maintenance of such systems.

The problems to be solved in each layer are different: it is not the same to transform a concept identifier from a format into another (e.g., by replacing its blank spaces with underscores) than to transform a set of logical restrictions into a disjoint decomposition of a concept. Therefore, each layer requires the use of different translation techniques.

In this section we describe the ODEDialect set of languages, which allows specifying translation decisions at the lexical (ODELex), syntax (ODESyntax), and semantic and pragmatic layers (ODESem). Only very specific input/output operations and complex transformations will have to be programmed with a generic programming language. The main advantage of this approach with respect to other existing approaches is that it allows concentrating on the transformations between knowledge models, rather than in other generic problems that arise when programming this type of information systems.

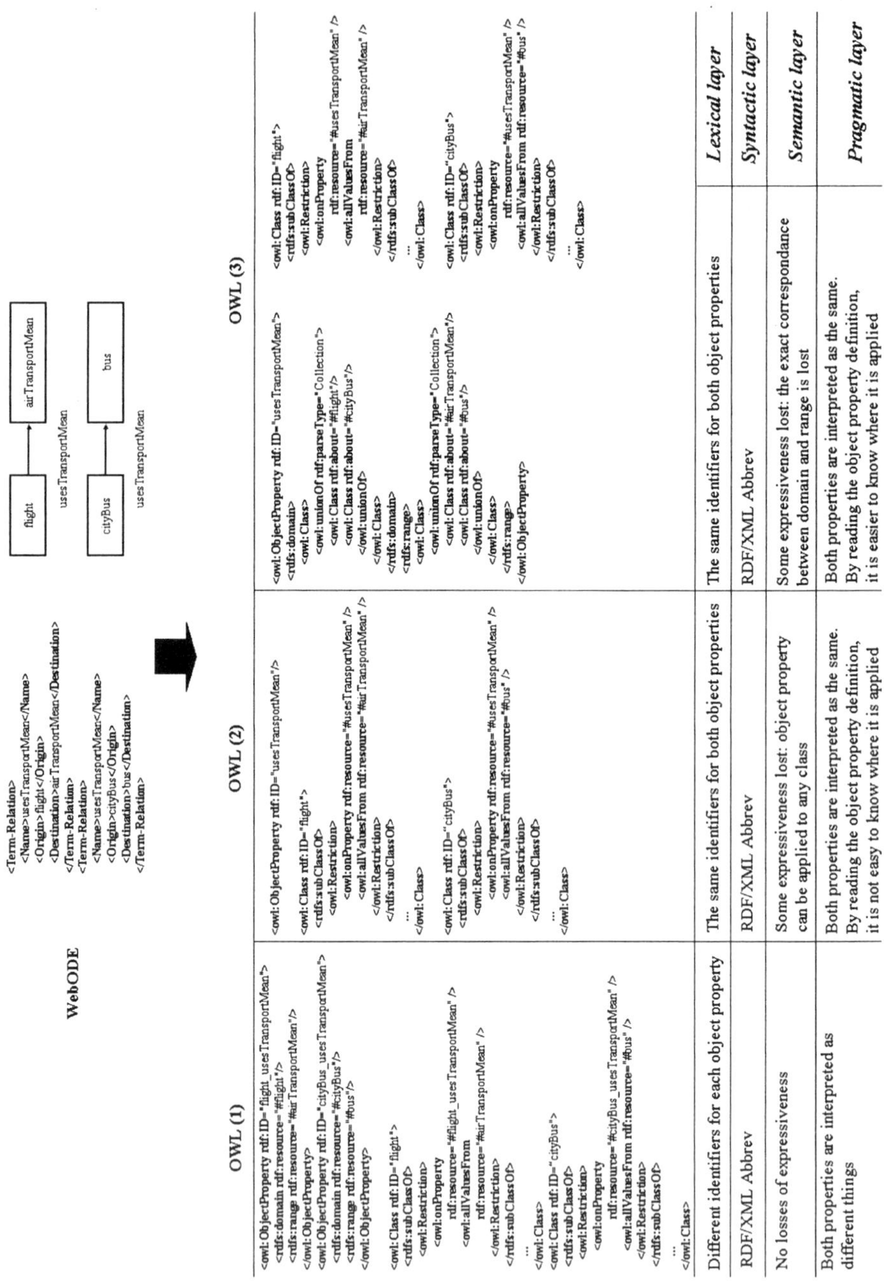

Figure 3.4. Example of translation decisions to be taken at several layers.

In the following subsections we will describe in detail the three languages that compose ODEDialect, whose BNF grammars are described in detail in annex III. These languages are related to each other as follows: transformations proposed at the semantic and pragmatic layers (with ODESem) use the transformations proposed at the syntax layer (with ODESyntax), which in its turn use the transformations proposed at the lexical layer (with ODELex).

3.3.1 Declarative Specification of Transformations at the Lexical Layer

As commented in section 3.2.1, the transformations at the lexical layer are mainly related to transforming ontology component identifiers (either because they contain characters in the source format that are illegal in the target one, or because of different naming conventions in the source and target formats, or because there are differences between the source and target formats with regard to the scope of identifiers) and pieces of text that are normally used to document ontology components. These problems are normally easy to handle, because we normally need to take into account the rules and conventions for creating identifiers and texts in both formats.

We propose to use the language ODELex to specify all the transformations of the lexical layer. This language is similar to lex [Lesk, 1975], a widely-used lexical analyzer for building compilers. While lex is aimed at building compilers, ODELex is optimized for building ontology translation systems, providing specific primitives related to the construction of this type of systems. We will now describe the main parts of an ODELex specification, using as an example the WebODE export service into OWL DL.

An ODELex specification is composed of three parts, as shown in the following derivation rule[28], which contain user code, declarations, and lexical rules. These parts are separated by the %% symbol. Besides, Java-style comments can be added at the beginning of the document, or inside the other parts, as will be seen later, in derivation rules 24, 25, and 26

(1) *ODELexDocument* :: {*comment*} **%%** [*userCode*] **%%** [*declarations*] **%%** [*lexRules*]

- ***User code***. The first part of an ODELex document contains the user code. Here users must include any Java functions used in the rest of the specification plus any Java import statements needed for these functions. These functions usually implement complex transformations of ontology component identifiers or pieces of text, or they are used as a kind of macro definitions for a sequence of transformations that have to be performed using standard functions from the Java API.

  (2) *userCode* :: {*comment*} **%(** *javaCode* **)%**

  The derivation that corresponds to the symbol *javaCode* is not included here, since it corresponds to the grammar used for any Java file, and hence can be found in other documents that deal with that programming language. In our example we have defined two Java functions:

  - *convertToURI*, which transforms a string value into a corresponding string value that is a valid URI.

  - *addNumber*, which adds the string "_1" to the identifier received as an input.

```
%(
import java.net.*;

private String convertToURI (String id){
   URI id_URI = new URI(URLEncoder.encode(id,"ISO-8859-1"))
   return id_URI.toString();
}
```

[28] *The following notation will be used to describe the derivation rules of the ODELex, ODESyntax and ODESem grammars: words in* italics *will be used for non-terminal symbols, words in* **bold** *font will be used for terminal symbols, alternatives will be represented with the | symbol, optional elements will be enclosed in square brackets* **[ ]***, iterations of 0 or more items will be enclosed in braces* **{ }***, and ranges of values will be enclosed in parenthesis and separated by hyphens* **(-)***.*

```
private String addNumber (String identifier){
  return (identifier + "_1");
}
)%
```

The definitions included in the user code part will be copied verbatim into the source file of the *LexicalMapper.java* file generated from this specification. In this part it is also possible to reference transformation functions from a lexer created with typical lexical analysis tools such as lex [Lesk, 1975; Levine et al., 1992], JLex[29] [Berk, 1997], etc.

- ***Declarations***. This part of an ODELex specification contains the declaration of which ontology components (both from the source format and from the target format) will be dealt with by the lexical transformation tool, and of which ontology components of the target format cannot overlap (which means that they cannot share the same identifiers as they share the same scope).

  (3) *declarations* :: {*comment* | *componentDecl* | *overlapDecl*}

  (4) *componentDecl* :: *idComponent* [**%transient**] [*scopeDecl*]

  (5) *scopeDecl* :: **%scope (** *idScope* {**,** *idScope*} **)**

  (6) *idScope* :: *idComponent* | *id*

  (7) *overlapDecl* :: **no-overlap (** *idComponent* **,** *idComponent* {**,** *idComponent*} **)**

  In the example below, the declaration part defines seven WebODE ontology components (concepts, instance attributes, class attributes, ad hoc relations, instances, bibliographic references, and formal axioms) and two types of values (values and documentation).

  Three of the WebODE components are not first class citizens of the ontology, since they are defined inside the scope of the others: instance and class attributes are defined inside the scope of concepts, and ad hoc relations are defined inside the scope of two concepts (their domain and range).

  Finally, the *%transient* keyword states that once that we have performed a transformation of the corresponding component, it is not worth storing the result of the transformation. In the example, this situation happens with attribute values and pieces of text used to document ontology components in both formats.

```
/* WebODE components */
WebODE.Concept
WebODE.InstanceAttribute %scope (WebODE.Concept)
WebODE.ClassAttribute %scope (WebODE.Concept)
WebODE.AdHocRelation %scope (WebODE.Concept,WebODE.Concept)
WebODE.Instance
WebODE.Reference
WebODE.Axiom
WebODE.Value %transient
WebODE.Documentation %transient
```

  With respect to OWL, it defines four ontology components (classes, object properties, datatype properties, instances) and two types of values (datatype values, and label and comments). It also states that the sets of identifiers of the four ontology components must be disjoint (they cannot overlap).

[29] *http://www.cs.princeton.edu/~appel/modern/java/JLex/*

```
/* OWL components */
OWL.Class
OWL.ObjectProperty
OWL.DatatypeProperty
OWL.Instance
OWL.DatatypeValue %transient
OWL.LabelComment %transient
no-overlap    (OWL.Class, OWL.ObjectProperty,
               OWL.DatatypeProperty, OWL.Instance)
```

This part of the code will be used to generate the file *LexicalTypes.java* that contains an interface with the components to be used in the lexical transformations. This interface will be used by the rest of lexical tools and by the tools from other layers.

- ***Lexical transformation rules***. This part of an ODELex specification contains the actual transformations that have to be performed for each ontology component of the source format to obtain its correspondence in the target format.

(8) *lexRules* :: {*lexRule*}

(9) *lexRule* :: *ruleHeader* CR *init* CR *table* CR *repeated* CR *overlap* CR

(10) *ruleHeader* :: **%** *idComponent* **IDENTIFIER** {*idComponent* **IDENTIFIER**}

As shown in rule 9, for each component specified in the lexical rule header the following information must be specified:

- INIT: it specifies the initial transformation to be performed, with an assignment in Java-style code, where $1 refers to the new value of the component identifier or piece of text and %1 refers to the original value.

  (11) *init* :: **INIT:**{*javaCode* }

- TABLE: if the component is not transient, it specifies the information to be stored so as to obtain it later either in the source format or in the target format.

  (12) *table* :: **TABLE:**{ *tableDecl* }

  (13) *tableDecl* :: **(** *tableColumn* **,** *tableColumn* **)**

  (14) *tableColumn* :: **[** *idComponent* **,** *numberPosition* {**,** *numberPosition*}**]**

  (15) *numberPosition* :: **%** *number* | **$** *number*

- REPEATED: if the component is not transient and cannot be repeated under certain circumstances, it specifies the alternative transformation to be made.

  (16) *repeated* :: **REPEATED:**{ *transformation* {**,** *transformation*} }

  (17) *transformation* :: *tablePatternColumn* **==>** {*javaCode* } |
  default **==>** {*javaCode* }

  (18) *tablePatternColumn* :: **[** *idComponent* **,** *numberPatternPosition*
  {**,** *numberPatternPosition*}**]**

  (19) *numberPatternPosition* :: **%** *number* | _

- OVERLAP: if the component is not transient and there cannot be overlaps in the target format, it specifies the transformation to be performed to the already generated identifier. This is repeated until there is no overlap.

  (20) *overlap* :: **OVERLAP:**{*javaCode* }

In the example below we propose to transform the identifier of a WebODE ad hoc relation into an identifier of an OWL ObjectProperty. The initial transformation consists in converting the identifier to a URI, with the function *convertToURI* specified above. Besides, we propose storing the ad hoc relation identifier and its two associated concept identifiers in the table *WebODE.AdHocRelation*, and the corresponding identifier obtained from the transformation in the table *OWL.ObjectProperty*, maintaining the corresponding links to each other. If the transformed OWL object property identifier already existed as an OWL object property identifier and if the WebODE ad hoc relation with the same ad hoc relation identifier and domain concept also existed, then we propose maintaining the identifier to be provided for the transformed object property. This identifier is obtained with the predefined function *GET*. The same applies if the same ad hoc relation identifier and range concept already existed. In another situation, a new identifier is created by adding the character "1" to the current transformed identifier. Finally, we propose adding a number to the OWL object property identifier until there is no collision with other class, datatype property, and instance identifiers (not with object properties).

```
%WebODE.AdHocRelation IDENTIFIER
        WebODE.Concept IDENTIFIER WebODE.Concept IDENTIFIER
  /* The 2nd and 3rd identifiers are of the domain and range
     concepts */
  INIT: {$1=convertToURI(%1)}
  TABLE:{([WebODE.AdHocRelation,%1,%2,%3],[OWL.ObjectProperty,$1])}
  REPEATED:
    {[WebODE.AdHocRelation,%1,%2,_] ==>
                    {$1=GET([WebODE.AdHocRelation,%1,%2,_])},
     [WebODE.AdHocRelation,%1,_,%3] ==>
                    {$1=GET([WebODE.AdHocRelation,%1,_,%3])},
     default ==> {$1=addNumber($1)}}
  OVERLAP: {$1=addNumber($1)}
```

This part of the ODELex specification will be used to generate most of the *LexicalMapper.java* file, which contains the lexical tools to be used by the tools generated by other layers to access the lexical information of each ontology component.

Finally, the following derivation rules are used for creating identifiers, Java-style comments, numbers and the end of line symbol. They have been used in the previous rules.

(21) *idComponent* :: *idFormat* **.** *id*

(22) *idFormat* :: **(A-Z){A-Z}**

(23) *id* :: **(A-Z,a-z){a-z,A-Z,0-9}**

(24) *comment* :: /* *textIncludingCR* */ | // *textWithoutCR*

(25) *textIncludingCR* :: **{a-z,A-Z,0-9,CR}**

(26) *textWithoutCR* :: **{a-z,A-Z,0-9}**

(27) *number* :: **(1-9){0-9}**

(28) *CR* :: **\n**

3.3.2 Declarative Specification of Transformations at the Syntactic Layer

One of our assumptions is that the source and the target formats of the transformations have their own Java APIs defined. Therefore, the transformations to be expressed in the syntactic layer are also simple, as occurred in the lexical layer. With regard to the source format, specifications at this layer describe the correspondence between each component and its accessors (either for the component itself, for all the components of a specific type, or for pieces of information of each component). With regard to the target format, specifications at this layer describe the correspondence between each component and its constructors, adding and updating methods as well as the accessors that might be needed. In this layer it is also specified the correspondence between the attribute datatypes of the source and the target formats.

The language ODESyntax specifyes the correspondences outlined above. As with ODELex, this language is based on another one available for building compilers, such as yacc [Johnson, 1975]. Any specification in ODESyntax is divided in several parts, described in detail below using examples that correspond to the WebODE export service to OWL DL.

The following rule shows that there are five parts: user code, declarations, accessors, constructor and updates, and datatype transformations.

(1) *ODESyntaxDocument* :: {*comment*} **%%** [*userCode*] **%%** [*declarations*]
%% [*accessDecls*] **%%** [*updateDecls*] **%%** [*datatype*]

- ***User code***. As with ODELex, the first part of an ODESyntax specification contains the user code, where all the auxiliary Java functions to be used in the rest of the specification are included. These functions usually implement complex syntactic transformations (e.g., of attribute datatypes) or they are used as a kind of macro definitions for transformations, accessors, updaters, etc., that have to be implemented as sequences of functions from the standard Java API or from the APIs of the source and target formats. The corresponding derivation rule is the same as in ODELex:

  (2) *userCode* :: {*comment*} **%(** *javaCode* **)%**

  The following examples, taken from the WebODE export service to OWL DL, show some of the auxiliary functions we have defined in this part:

  - *getConcepts*, which receives as an input an ontology name and returns all the concepts in the WebODE ontology. This function is defined here because the current WebODE ontology access API does not provide such a method.

  - *addComment*, which receives the class where the comment must be added and the text of the comment. This function is defined here because in the Jena API (used to generate the target OWL ontology) the language in which the comment text is available must be specified. This function ensures that this language is set to null. As we will see further on, this could have been omitted since this function is used mostly as a macro.

  - *removeAllSuperclasses*, which receives an OWL class and removes all the references to the class superclasses. This function is defined here because the Jena API does not provide a specific function for performing this action, and it will be used in one of the following parts of the ODESyntax specification.

```
%(
//Import statements for the source format
import es.upm.fi.dia.ontology.webode.service.*;
//Import statements for the target format
import com.hp.hpl.jena.ontology.*;
```

```
private Concept[] getConcepts(String ontology){
  return (Concept[] (ode.getTerms
              (ontology, new int [] {TermTypes.CONCEPT})));
}

private void addComment(OntClass class, String commentText) {
  class.addComment(commentText,null);
       //the second argument is used for specifying the language
}

private void removeAllSuperclasses(OntClass class){
  ExtendedIterator iter = class.listSuperClasses();
  if (iter!=null){
       while (iter.hasNext()){
            class.removeSuperClass((OntClass)iter.next());
       }
  }
}
...
)%
```

The definitions included in the user code part will be copied verbatim into the source file of the *SyntaxMapper.java* file generated from this specification. We have also considered the possibility of referencing transformation functions from a syntax analyzer created with typical syntax analysis tools such as yacc [Johnson, 1975; Levine et al., 1992], JCup[30] [Hudson, 1999], etc.

- ***Declarations***. As in ODELex, this part of an ODESyntax specification contains the declaration of which ontology components will be dealt with in the specification. This component list does not need to contain the same components than the ODELex, since it has a different purpose (syntactic transformations instead of lexical ones). Besides, it does not have to consider whether a component is transient or not, nor whether there can be overlap or not with other components, since these problems are already solved by the lexical layer specification. The following rules are used to create this declaration part of the ODESyntax document:

  (3) *declarations* :: {*comment* | *namespaceDecl* | *componentDecl* }

  (4) *namespaceDecl* :: **%NAMESPACE** *id javaPackage* ;

  (5) *componentDecl* :: *idComponent* [*scopeDecl*] **:** *javaClassID* **CR**

  (6) *scopeDecl* :: **%scope (** *idComponent* {**,** *idComponent*} **)**

  The ODESyntax component list is usually based on the knowledge models of the source and target formats. Furthermore, it usually corresponds to their APIs. If there is a strong correspondence between the format knowledge model and its API (either of the source or of the target format), the transformations to be specified in ODESyntax are quite straightforward. If not, the transformations are more complex and more effort is needed to construct the ODESyntax specification.

  The declaration part also includes a list of namespaces, which is used to abbreviate long Java packages in the rest of the specification. To refer to these namespaces, the corresponding namespace identifier must be placed between square brackets (e.g., *[ode]* to refer to *es.upm.fi.dia.ontology.webode.service.*).

  The declaration part of the example below defines two namespaces (*ode* and *jenaOnt*), which correspond to the packages where the knowledge models of the source and

[30] *http://www.cs.princeton.edu/~appel/modern/java/CUP/*

target formats are defined. This part also defines the ontology components from the source and target formats that will be used for the syntactic transformations, together with their scope, in case that they depend on another components, and with their corresponding Java class or interface. In the case that a component does not have an interface or class defined for it in the format's API, we should create one in the user code part or in an external file, and make references to it from this specification.

```
%NAMESPACE ode es.upm.fi.dia.ontology.webode.service.;
%NAMESPACE jenaOnt com.hp.hpl.jena.ontology.;

/* WebODE components */
WebODE.Ontology                  :[ode]OntologyDescriptor
WebODE.Concept
  %scope (WebODE.Ontology)       :[ode]Concept
WebODE Group
  %scope (WebODE.Ontology)       :[ode]Group
WebODE.InstanceAttribute
  %scope (WebODE.Concept,
          WebODE.Ontology)       :[ode]InstanceAttributeDescriptor
WebODE.ClassAttribute
  %scope (WebODE.Concept)        :[ode]ClassAttributeDescriptor
WebODE.AdHocRelation
  %scope (WebODE.Concept,
          WebODE.Concept)        :[ode]TermRelation
WebODE.Reference
  %scope (WebODE.Ontology)       :[ode]ReferenceDescriptor
WebODE.Axiom
  %scope (WebODE.Ontology)       :[ode]FormulaDescriptor
WebODE.Instance
  %scope (WebODE.Ontology,
          WebODE.InstanceSet)    :[ode]Instance
WebODE.InstanceSet
  %scope (WebODE.Ontology)       :[ode]InstanceSet

/* OWL components */
OWL.Ontology                :[jenaOnt]Ontology
OWL.Class                   :[jenaOnt]OntClass
OWL.ObjectProperty          :[jenaOnt]ObjectProperty
OWL.DatatypeProperty        :[jenaOnt]DatatypeProperty
OWL.Instance                :[jenaOnt]Individual
```

Unlike in ODELex, the declaration part of an ODESyntax specification must include all the components that will be managed by the syntax transformations.

- ***Accessor methods***. For each ontology component of the source and target formats that has been declared in the previous piece of code, this part of an ODESyntax specification may declare the methods to be used for the following purposes:
    - To access all the ontology components of a specific type (e.g., a method that retrieves all the concepts of an ontology).
    - To access a specific ontology component of a specific type (e.g., a method that retrieves a specific concept of an ontology, given its identifier).
    - To access different pieces of information of the ontology component (e.g., methods or properties to access a concept identifier, a concept description, the superclasses of a concept, etc.).

The following rules show the grammar for these methods:

(7) *accessDecls* :: {*accessDecl*}

(8) *accessDecl* :: *header* **CR** [*all* **CR**] [*individual* **CR**] [*information* **CR**]

(9) *header* :: **%** *idComponent* **IDENTIFIER** {*idComponent* **IDENTIFIER**}

(10) *all* :: **ALL:{** *functionDecl* {**;** *functionDecl* } **}**

(11) *individual* :: **INDIVIDUAL:{** *functionDecl* {**;** *functionDecl* } **}**

(12) *functionDecl* :: *number* **:** *id* **(** *parameters* **)** **:** *javaClassID array*

(13) *parameters* :: **%** *number* { **,** **%** *number* } | λ

(14) *array* :: **[]** | λ

(15) *information* :: **INFORMATION:{** *informDecl* {**;** *informDecl* } **}**

(16) *informDecl* :: *id* **:** *id* [**(** *parameters* **)**] **:** *javaClassID array*

As shown in the previous rules, the first group of accessors will be included in the *ALL* keyword, the second in the *INDIVIDUAL* keyword, and the third in the *INFORMATION* keyword. For each method in the first and second groups, we will indicate a number that identifies the method (as there can be different methods with the same purpose), the method name and parameters, and the object that it returns. For the third group, we specify the piece of information identifier (which determines how we will access this information from the semantic and pragmatic layers), the property or method to be used to access to that information given a specific object of that type, and the datatype.

The following example shows the declaration corresponding to an ontology component of the source format: a WebODE instance attribute. It shows that instance attributes are defined inside the scope of an ontology and of a concept. There are two methods that allow accessing all the instance attributes of a concept in an ontology: the first one is used to access the instance attributes that are defined explicitly in that concept, and the second returns also those inherited through the concept taxonomy. Both of them return an array of objects of the class *InstanceAttributeDescriptor*.

There is one method to get a specific instance attribute, whose input is the ontology name, the concept name, and the attribute name.

Finally, the following information can be accessed from an instance attribute: the concept to which it belongs, the attribute name, the attribute description, its type, its maximum and minimum cardinality, its maximum and minimum value, and the set of explicit values. This information is accessed with properties of the Java class *InstanceAttributeDescriptor*, except for the attribute type, which is accessed with an ad hoc function defined in the user code part.

```
%WebODE.InstanceAttribute IDENTIFIER
    WebODE.Concept IDENTIFIER
    WebODE.Ontology IDENTIFIER
ALL:
{1:getInstanceAttributes(%3,%2):[ode]InstanceAttributeDescriptor[];
         //gets instance attributes defined locally to the concept
 2:getInstanceAttributes(%3,%2,true)
                                :[ode]InstanceAttributeDescriptor[]
         //gets also inherited instance attributes
  }
INDIVIDUAL:
{1:getInstanceAttribute(%3,%2,%1):[ode]InstanceAttributeDescriptor}
```

```
INFORMATION:
 {concept      :termName                      :String;
  Name         :name                          :String;
  Description  :description                   :String;
  Type         :getValueTypeName(valueType)   :String;
  MaxCard      :maxCardinality                :int;
  MinCard      :minCardinality                :int;
  MaxValue     :maxValue                      :float;
  MinValue     :minValue                      :float;
  Values       :values                        :String[]}
```

The following example shows the declaration that corresponds to an OWL class (an ontology component of the target format). It shows that OWL classes are not in the scope of other components, that there is a method that lists all the classes of an ontology, that there is also a method to access a specific class given its identifier, and that we can access to the class name, to its description and to its superclasses. In some of these cases a *java.util.Iterator* is returned.

```
%OWL.Class IDENTIFIER
ALL:            {1:listClasses()          :java.util.Iterator}
INDIVIDUAL:     {1:getOntClass(%1)        :[jenaOnt]OntClass}
INFORMATION:
 {name          :getURI()                 :String;
  description   :listComments(null)       :java.util.Iterator;
  subclassOf    :listSuperClasses()       :java.util.Iterator}
```

As commented in the declaration part, if a specific method or property that we want to specify in this part is not defined in the ontology access API of a format, we can define them either in the user code part of the ODESyntax specification or in a separate file that will extend the current API.

- ***Constructor and update methods***. For each ontology component of the target format that has been declared in the declaration part, this part of an ODESyntax specification may declare the methods that will be used for the following purposes:
  - To create the ontology component in the target ontology (e.g., a constructor or a method that creates an OWL class) we use the keyword *CREATE*.
  - To remove the ontology component from the target ontology (e.g., a method that removes a class from an OWL ontology) we use the keyword *REMOVE*.
  - To add information about the ontology component (e.g., the method or property to be used to add information about the class documentation, the class superclasses, etc.) we use the keyword *ADD*.
  - To remove all the information about a specific piece of information of the ontology component (e.g., the method or property to be used to remove all the class documentations, all the class superclasses, etc.) we use the keyword *REMOVEALL*.
  - To remove a value from a specific piece of information of the ontology component (e.g., the method or property to be used to remove a specific class documentation, a specific class superclass, etc.) we use the keyword *REMOVEINDIVIDUAL*.

The following derivation rules show the syntax to be used to declare these constructors and update methods:

(17) *updateDecls* :: {*updateDecl*}

(18) *updateDecl* :: *header* **CR** [*create* **CR**] [*remove* **CR**] [*add* **CR**]
[*removeall* **CR**] [*removeindividual* **CR**]

(19) *create* :: **CREATE:{** *createremDecl* {**;** *createremDecl* } **}**

(20) *remove* :: **REMOVE:{** *createremDecl* {**;** *createremDecl* } **}**

(21) *createremDecl* :: *number* **:** *id* **(** *parameters* **)**

(22) *add* :: **ADD:{** *addremDecl* {**;** *addremDecl* } **}**

(23) *removeall* :: **REMOVEALL:{** *addremDecl* {**;** *addremDecl* } **}**

(24) *removeindividual* :: **REMOVEINDIVIDUAL:{** *addremDecl* {**;** *addremDecl* } **}**

(25) *addremDecl* :: *id* **:** *id* **(** *parameters* **)**

For each method in the first and second groups, we will indicate a number that identifies the method (as there can be different methods with the same purpose), the method name and parameters. For the rest of the groups, we specify the piece of information identifier (which determines how we will access this information from the semantic and pragmatic layers), and the property or method to use to add, remove all, and remove one of the value(s) of that piece of information, respectively. Not all the pieces of information must be specified in all the cases but only those used by the transformations in the semantic and pragmatic layers.

The following example shows the declaration corresponding to an OWL class. It shows that there is one method that allows creating classes in the target ontology, *createClass*, which receives the identifier of the class as an input. It also defines the methods that can be used to add a natural language description to the class and to remove all the descriptions, and the methods to use to add a superclass, to remove all the class superclasses, and to remove a specific superclass. The %1 parameter refers to the OWL class identifier, and the $1 in the parameter means that the value of this parameter (the actual description and the class identifier) will be provided by the semantic or pragmatic layers in the first order. We will see how to define this information in the semantic and pragmatic transformation layers.

```
%OWL.Class IDENTIFIER
CREATE:          {1:createClass(%1)}
ADD:             {description      :addComment(%1,$1);
                  subclassOf       :addSuperClass(createClass($1))}
REMOVEALL:       {description      :removeAllComments(%1);
                  subclassOf       :removeAllSuperclasses(%1)}
REMOVEINDIVIDUAL:{subclassOf       :removeSuperClass(createClass($1))}
```

As we have commented for other parts of the specification, if a specific method or property used in this part is not defined in the ontology access API of a format, we can define them either in the user code part of the ODESyntax specification or in a separate file that will extend the current API.

- ***Datatype transformations***. This part of an ODESyntax specification contains the transformations that have to be made to the attribute datatypes that appear in the source format so as to transform them into the target format. This specific feature, which may have been included in the previous part of the specification (constructors and updater methods), aims to make the specification of these common transformations easier.

  The following derivation rules are defined in the ODESyntax grammar to deal with this type of transformations:

  (26) *datatype* :: {*datatypeTransf*}

  (27) *datatypeTransf* :: **"** *datatypeID* **" : "** *datatypeID* **" ;** |
  default %1 : (*datatypeID* | **%1** | **{** *javaCode* **}**)

The following example shows how to specify datatype transformations from WebODE to OWL DL. Before the ':' symbol, we specify the String term used to identify the type in the source format. After the ':' symbol, we specify the correspondence for each datatype of the source format in the target format (in this example, all of them are XML Schema datatypes, since OWL DL only allows them to specify datatypes). The transformations will be checked sequentially, according to the order specified here. Besides, the "default" keyword can be used in the last line to specify any other kind of datatype that could be found.

```
/* Datatype transformations */
"boolean":   "http://www.w3.org/2001/XMLSchema#boolean";
"cardinal":  "http://www.w3.org/2001/XMLSchema#nonNegativeInteger";
"integer":   "http://www.w3.org/2001/XMLSchema#integer";
"float":     "http://www.w3.org/2001/XMLSchema#float";
"string":    "http://www.w3.org/2001/XMLSchema#string";
"date":      "http://www.w3.org/2001/XMLSchema#date";
"range":     "http://www.w3.org/2001/XMLSchema#float";
"URL":       "http://www.w3.org/2001/XMLSchema#anyURI";
default %1: %1;
```

Finally, there are some non-terminal symbols that have been used by the previous rules of the ODESyntax grammar and whose derivation rules have not appeared yet. Besides the rules of this type that were defined for ODELex, we have the following additional ones:

(36) *javaClassID* :: **[** *id* **]** *id*

(37) *javaPackage* :: *id* **.** { *id* **.**}

(38) *datatypeID* :: {**a-z,A-Z,0-9,:,/,#**}

3.3.3 Declarative Specification of Transformations at the Semantic and Pragmatic Layers

In the previous sections we have described how to specify declaratively the transformations to be made in the lexical and syntactic layers. The main objective of both transformation layers is to abstract the low-level details of the source and target formats (their syntax specific features, the restrictions and naming conventions of ontology component identifiers, etc.), to allow specifying the semantic and pragmatic transformations at a higher abstraction level.

In our proposal, we have considered the assumption that the problems to be solved in the semantic and pragmatic layers are the most important (and complex) ones, since they decide which transformations have to be performed by the ontology translation system. Hence the importance of abstracting low-level details of the source and target formats to allow knowledge engineers to focus on the transformations between their knowledge models.

As described in section 3.2.3, the problems to be solved in the semantic layer are mainly related to complex transformations of expressions that go beyond the simple limits of syntax and whose general aim is usually to preserve the meaning of the knowledge transformed. Some examples of such transformations are:

- Transform a component of the source format into several components in the target format. For instance, an OWL value restriction is transformed into a WebODE instance attribute and an explicit value assignment to that instance attribute.
- Transform a set of components of the source format into one component in the target format. For instance, a set of OWL *disjointWith* expressions and *subclass of* relationships are transformed into a WebODE disjoint decomposition.

- Transform a component of the source format into different components of the target format depending on some conditions. For instance, an RDF property must be transformed into a WebODE ad hoc relation if its range is an RDF class, and to a WebODE instance attribute if its range is a literal or an XML Schema datatype.

As described in section 3.2.4, the problems to be solved in the pragmatic layer are those that permit human users and ontology-based applications to notice as less differences as possible in the ontologies in the original and target formats. Examples of such transformations are:

- *Pre-processing transformations*. These usually consist in the creation of predefined ontology components in the target format to facilitate the transformation of other ontology components during the semantic processing. For example, creating the metaclass *:WebODEConcept* in Protégé-2000 to store additional information about the ontology concepts being transformed from WebODE to Protégé-2000
- *Post-processing transformations*. These usually consist in transforming sets of expressions in the target format, which have been created as a result of the semantic transformations, into more legible (and usually equivalent) syntactic constructs in the target format. Some examples of such transformations are: transforming a set of WebODE formal axioms that define that several concepts are disjoint to each other into a WebODE concept group; transforming a domain of an OWL object property of the form `C1 U C2 U ... U Cn` into a more general concept that subsumes the union of that concept; etc.
- *In-processing transformations*. Pragmatic decisions can also be taken during the processing of individual ontology components of the source format. These transformations differ from the semantic ones in the fact that they do not change the semantics of the knowledge transformed, but the way in which it can be interpreted by humans. Examples of such decisions are: whether to transform an RDF property without range into a WebODE instance attribute with type *String*, into a WebODE ad hoc relation with the ontology root concept as the range, or into both; which name should be assigned to the WebODE formal axiom derived from an OWL complete class definition; which name should be assigned to the WebODE anonymous class obtained from an OWL union of classes; etc.
- *Other transformations*. In this group we include any other transformation and decision to be made during the ontology translation process for pragmatic reasons, and that cannot be easily classified in the previous groups. For instance, hiding in the Protégé-2000 user interface the additional ontology components used to transform a WebODE ontology, so that users cannot find differences with the standard Protégé-2000 knowledge model.

The translation decisions in both layers will be specified with the same declarative language: ODESem. As we did with the other two languages presented in this chapter (ODELex and ODESyntax), we will now describe the parts in which this language is divided. The first derivation rule of the grammar shows that an ODESem specification is divided into three parts: user defined code, declarations and semantic and pragmatic rules:

(1) *ODESemDocument* :: {*comment*} **%%** [*userCode*] **%%** [*declarations*] **%%** [*semRules*]

- ***User code***. As with the other two languages, the first part of an ODESem specification contains the user code, where all the auxiliary Java functions to be used in the rest of the specification are included. As we have commented above, there might be a need for performing complex transformations that might not be easily represented with the primitives used in other parts of the specification. In this case, this user defined functions can be used from those parts. The grammar rule used for the user code part of an ODESem specification is like the ones used in the other two languages:

(2) *userCode* :: {*comment*} **%(** *javaCode* **)%**

The following examples, taken from the WebODE export service to OWL DL, show some auxiliary functions defined in this part:

- *obtainDatatypes* and *obtainDomains*, which receive the identifier of an OWL datatype property as an input and return all the datatypes and domains associated to it, as they were stored in the lexical transformation mapping tools created from the ODELex specification. These functions are provided as shortcuts for the use of the predefined lexical function *obtainDistinctSourceParametersFromTargetId.*
- *obtainDatatype* and *obtainDomain*, which are similar to the previous ones, but return only one datatype and domain, respectively. These functions are used when the datatype property has only one datatype or range.
- *allDatatypesEqual* and *allDomainsEqual*, which receive the identifier of an OWL datatype property as an input and return true if it has only one datatype, and one domain or not, respectively. These functions are also shortcuts for the use of the predefined lexical function *obtainDistinctSourceParametersFromTargetId* and the check of the return value length.

```
private String[] obtainDatatypes (String propID){
  return obtainDistinctSourceParameterFromTargetID
        (LexicalMapper.OWL_DatatypeProperty,propID,2);
}
private String obtainDatatype (String propID){
  return obtainDistinctSourceParameterFromTargetID
        (LexicalMapper.OWL_DatatypeProperty,propID,2)[0];
}
private String[] obtainDomains (String propID){
  return obtainDistinctSourceParameterFromTargetID
        (LexicalMapper.OWL_DatatypeProperty,propID,1);
}
private String[] obtainDomain (String propID){
  return obtainDistinctSourceParameterFromTargetID
        (LexicalMapper.OWL_DatatypeProperty,propID,1)[0];
}
private boolean allDatatypesEqual (String propID){
  return (obtainDistinctSourceParameterFromTargetID
        (LexicalMapper.OWL_DatatypeProperty,propID,2).length<=1);
}
private boolean allDomainsEqual (String propID){
return (obtainDistinctSourceParameterFromTargetID
        (LexicalMapper.OWL_DatatypeProperty,propID,1).length<=1);
}
```

As with the other two languages, the user code part will be copied verbatim into the source file of the *SemMapper.java* file generated from this specification.

- ***Semantic and pragmatic transformation rule declarations and processing order***. This part of an ODESem specification contains the declaration of the transformation rules that will be defined later, and the order in which they have to be processed. Unlike in the rest of declarative specifications, where the order of the definitions is not relevant, in this case the processing order of the semantic and pragmatic transformations might be relevant and hence it is considered in this specification.

The following rules of the ODESem grammar define how these rules and their processing order are defined:

(3) *declarations* :: {*comment* | *ruleDecl* }

(4) *ruleDecl* :: *number* **: %** *id* **;**

The following piece of code shows these declarations for the WebODE export service into OWL DL. This export service does not need to execute pre-processing rules. The rules 1 to 7 are in charge of the semantic and pragmatic transformations of the components found in the source format (the WebODE ontology). As we can infer from the rule names, the ontology translation system will first add general information about the ontology (ontology container), the classes, the object properties, the disjoint and exhaustive decompositions, and the ontology instances. Finally, three pragmatic post-processing transformations will be performed to remove redundant domains in OWL datatype property definitions and redundant domains and ranges in OWL object property definitions.

```
/* Semantic and pragmatic transformation rule declaration,
   and processing sequence */
1: %AddOntologyContainer;
2: %AddClasses;
3: %AddObjectProperties;
4: %AddDisjointDecompositions;
5: %AddExhaustiveDecompositions;
6: %AddInstances;
7: %PostProcessing_RemoveDPRedundantDomains;
8: %PostProcessing_RemoveOPRedundantDomains;
9: %PostProcessing_RemoveOPRedundantRanges;
```

- ***Semantic and pragmatic transformation rules***. The last part of an ODESem specification contains the rules to be applied in order to transform the ontology components in the source format into the corresponding ontology components in the target format. This part of the specification must contain at least the rules declared previously plus any other auxiliary rules that can be called from these ones.

  A semantic and/or pragmatic transformation rule is referred to with an identifier, which is preceded by the symbol '%'. This is what is called header in the ODESem grammar, as shown below:

  (5) *semRules* :: {*semRule* | *comment*}

  (6) *semRule* :: *header* **CR** *lhs* **-->** **{** *rhs* **}**

  (7) *header* :: **%** *id*

  Besides, , as shown in the previous derivation grammar rule, a transformation rule is define with two parts: the left hand side (LHS) and the right hand side (RHS):

  - The LHS (Left Hand Side) of the rule, aka antecedent, contains the information needed to trigger the rule, which can be either the source ontology component to be transformed or a target component to be modified. In both cases, the antecedent is defined with the ontology component type, as defined in the ODESyntax specification, and with an identifier that will be used to refer to the specific component in the RHS (Right Hand Side) of the rule. If no information is needed to trigger the rule, the keyword *NULL* must be used.

    (8) *lhs* :: *idComponent id* | **NULL**

- The RHS of the rule, aka consequent, contains the sequence of actions that have to be performed to obtain the corresponding ontology component(s) in the target format.

  The following rule of the ODESem grammar defines the set of actions that can be performed in the RHS of the transformation rule:

  (9) *rhs* :: { *create* | *add* | *remove* | *removeall* | *exec* | *ifThen* | *forEach*
  | *error* | *assign* | *functionCall*} **;**

  These actions can be grouped in three types: actions that create new ontology components in the target format, and add or remove components or information; actions that specify the control flow of the translation system; and general actions used to throw error messages, assign values to variables or call other functions, either predefined or defined by the user.

  Let us start with the first group of actions, whose corresponding piece of grammar is shown below:

  (16) *create* :: **CREATE (** *idComponent* **,** *number* **,** *var* {**,** *var*}**)**

  (17) *add* :: **ADD (** *id* **,** *id* **,** (*create* | *var* | *getComponents*) **)**

  (18) *remove* :: **REMOVE (** *id* **,** *id* **,** *var* **)**

  (19) *removeall* :: **REMOVEALL (** *id* **,** *id* **)**

  - CREATE. It creates (and returns) an ontology component in the target ontology. As input parameters this action receives the ontology component type to be created, the number of the specific constructor to be used, and the rest of parameters needed to create the ontology component. All the information needed (the ontology component type, the number of the specific constructor and the number and order of the additional input parameters) must follow the restrictions coded in the ODESyntax specification.
  - ADD. It adds one or several values to a specific property of an ontology component of the target ontology. The ontology component, the property and the value(s) are specified as input parameters.
  - REMOVE. It removes a value from a specific property of an ontology component of the target ontology. The ontology component, the property and the value to be removed are specified as input parameters.
  - REMOVEALL. It removes all the values from a specific property of an ontology component of the target ontology. The ontology component and the property are specified as input parameters.

  The actions specified in the consequent of a transformation rule are executed sequentially. Besides, the following control flow structures can be used:

  (20) *exec* :: **EXEC (%** *id* **,** *var* **)**

  (13) *ifThen* :: **if (** *condition* **)** [{] *rhs* [}] **else** [{] *rhs* [}]

  (14) *condition* :: *javaComparison* | *functionCall*

  (15) *forEach* :: **forEach** *id* **IN** *var* [{] *rhs* [}]

  - EXEC. It starts the execution of a rule with the set of parameters that match its antecedent.

- If *condition* {*rhs*} else {*rhs*}. It specifies the set of actions to be performed if the condition specified is evaluated as true (*then* body), and, optionally, the set of actions to be performed if the condition specified is evaluated as false (*else* body).
- ForEach id IN *var* {*rhs*}. It specifies the set of actions to be performed for each ontology component inside the multiple-valued variable.

Finally, any variable assignments can be used using the form *var* = *value*, and the predefined functions *GETCOMPONENT* and *GETALLCOMPONENTS* can be used to obtain a specific component or all the components of either the source or the target format (with the parameters specified in the ODESyntax specification). The *ERROR* function can be used in cases where the options that allow executing it are not allowed. These actions are considered in the following ODESem grammar rules:

(10) *assign* :: *id* = { *create* | *functionCall* | *getComponents*}

(11) *functionCall* :: *id* **(** *parameters* **)**

(12) *parameters* :: *id* { **,** *id* } | λ

(24) *getComponents* :: **GETCOMPONENT (** *idComponent* **,** *id* **)** |
GETALLCOMPONENTS (*idComponent* **,** *id* **)**

Below we provide the code of some transformation rules of the WebODE export service into OWL DL, specifically those that transform WebODE concepts and their instance attributes in OWL classes and datatype properties.

The first rule (*AddClasses*) appeared in the declaration and processing order part of the specification. For each concept defined in WebODE, it creates an OWL class with the concept name, it adds a natural language description, in case that it exists and that the concept is not an imported term from another ontology, and it states that it is a subclass of the parent concepts, as specified in the source format. Finally, for each instance attribute of the concept, the rule *ADDInstanceAttributes* is triggered.

```
%AddClasses
WebODE.Concept concept -->
  {C = CREATE(OWL.Class,1,concept.name);
   if (concept.description != null && !concept.isImported)
        ADD(C,description,concept.description);
   ADD(C,subClassOf,concept.parentConcepts);
   forEach ia IN concept.instanceAttributes
        EXEC(%AddInstanceAttributes,WebODE.InstanceAttribute,ia);
  }
```

The second rule (*AddInstanceAttributes*) did not appear in the declaration and processing order section of the specification, hence it is considered as an auxiliary rule. It creates an OWL datatype property from a WebODE instance attribute; besides, it implements a decision tree that depends on whether there are several instance attributes in WebODE that produce the same OWL identifier or not, and in the first case, whether those instance attributes have the same datatype associated or not. Depending on these conditions, the rules *AddInstanceAttributes_1* or *AddInstanceAttributes_2* will be triggered, or an error will be obtained.

```
%AddInstanceAttributes
WebODE.InstanceAttribute instAttr -->
  {P = CREATE(OWL.DatatypeProperty,1,propertyID);
   if (targetIDhasSeveralSources (WebODE.InstanceAttribute,
                      instAttr.name,instAttr.concept,instAttr.type) {
        if (allDatatypesEqual (WebODE.InstanceAttribute,
```

```
                instAttr.name,instAttr.concept,instAttr.type))
            EXEC(%AddInstanceAttributes_1,P);
        else  ERROR("Datatype property with multiple datatypes");
  }else  EXEC(%AddInstanceAttributes_2,P);
  }
```

Finally, the last two auxiliary rules are in charge of updating the information that corresponds to the datatype property created by the previous one. The first one (*AddInstanceAttributes_1*) is used when there are several instance attributes in WebODE that produce the same identifier, since they share the same datatype. This rule creates the union of all the concepts where those instance attributes are defined, and set the union as the domain of the datatype property. It also states that the range of the property created is the datatype of all those instance attributes. Finally, for each OWL class in the domain of the property it creates an OWL *AllValuesFrom* restriction and the corresponding minimum and maximum cardinality restrictions, and it attaches them as *subclass of* restrictions of the class. The second rule (*AddInstanceAttributes_2*) is used when there is only one instance attribute that produces that datatype property identifier. In this case, the rule establishes the domain and range of the property and adds OWL *AllValuesFrom* and maximum and minimum cardinality restrictions to the corresponding domain class.

```
%AddInstanceAttributes_1
OWL.DatatypeProperty P -->
  {domains = obtainDomains(P);
   ADD(P,domain,CREATE(OWL.UnionOf,1,domains));
   ADD(P,range,obtainDatatype(P.name));
   forEach d IN domains {
      D = GETCOMPONENT(OWL.Class,d);
      ADD(D,subClassOf,
          CREATE(OWL.AllValuesFrom,1,P,obtainDatatype(P.name)));
      if (instAttr.minCard!=0)
          ADD(D,subClassOf,
              CREATE(OWL.MinCardRestriction,1,P,instAttr.minCard));
      if (instAttr.maxCard!=-1)
          ADD(D,subClassOf,
              CREATE(OWL.MaxCardRestriction,1,P,instAttr.maxCard));
   }
  }

%AddInstanceAttributes_2
OWL.DatatypeProperty P -->
  {ADD(P,domain,obtainDomain(P.name));
   ADD(P,range,obtainDatatype(P.name));
   D = GETCOMPONENT(OWL.Class,d);
   ADD(D,subClassOf,
       CREATE(OWL.AllValuesFrom,1,P, obtainDatatype(P.name)));
   if (instAttr.minCard!=0)
       ADD(D,subClassOf,
           CREATE(OWL.MinCardRestriction,1,P,instAttr.minCard));
   if (instAttr.maxCard!=-1)
       ADD(D,subClassOf,
           CREATE(OWL.MaxCardRestriction,1,P,instAttr.maxCard));
  }
```

Finally, we will show a transformation rule that corresponds to the pragmatic post-processing of datatype properties to remove the redundant domains. This transformation rule consists in checking whether the domain of a datatype property is an OWL union of classes. Then, if any of the classes in that union is already a subclass of any of the other concepts in the union, the class can be removed because it is already included in the domain.

```
%PostProcessing_RemoveDPRedundantDomains
OWL.DatatypeProperty P -->
   {forEach U in P.domain {
         if (U.isUnionOf)
               forEach D in U.classes
                     forEach E in U.classes
                           if (E.isSubclassOf(D)) REMOVE(U,class,E)
   }
```

3.4 A Method for Building an Ontology Translation System

This section presents a method for developing ontology translation systems taking into account the two restrictions described in sections 3.2 and 3.3: (1) that transformations between two formats can be designed and implemented in four different layers: lexical, syntax, semantic and pragmatic; and (2) that the approach for building ontology translation systems must be declarative, so that they are easier to build and maintain.

The method consists of four activities: feasibility study, analysis of source and target formats, design of the translation system, and implementation of the translation system. Activities are divided into tasks that can be performed by different sets of people and with different techniques.

The method recommends the development of ontology translation systems following an iterative life cycle. It proposes identifying a first set of expressions that can be easily translated from one format into another so that the first version of the ontology translation system can be quickly developed and tested; then it proposes refining the transformations performed, analyzing more complex expressions and designing and implementing their transformations. The reason for such a recommendation is that developing an ontology translation system is usually a complex task that requires taking into account too many aspects of the source and target formats, and many different types of decisions on how to perform specific translations. In this sense, an iterative life cycle ensures that complex translation problems are tackled once that the developers have a better knowledge of the source and target formats and that they have tested simpler translations performed with earlier versions of the software produced.

The feasibility activity is performed at the beginning of the development process. If the study recommends developing the translation system then, for each cycle, the other three activities are performed sequentially. Developers can always go back to previous activities with the feedback provided by the subsequent ones, as shown in figure 3.5.

As a summary, table 3.2 lists the activities that the method proposes and the tasks to be performed inside each activity. The design and implementation activities take into account the four translation layers described in the previous sections.

The method does not put special emphasis on other activities usually related to software development, either specific to the software development process such as deployment and maintenance, or related to support activities such as quality assurance, project management and configuration management. Nor does it emphasize other tasks usually performed during the feasibility study, analysis, design, and implementation activities of general software development. It only describes those specifically related to the development of ontology translation systems, and recommends performing such additional activities and tasks.

Now we describe in detail each of the four activities proposed. Activities are described with the same structure: we describe first the overall objectives of the activity; then the organization of the activity into tasks and the order in which they should be accomplished; and finally the activity inputs and outputs, the participants involved in it, and the techniques

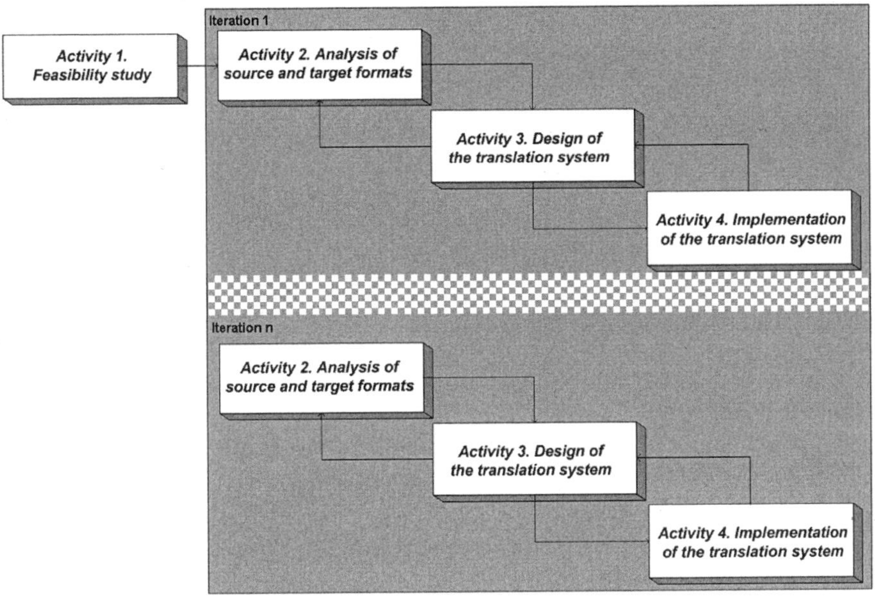

Figure 3.5. Proposed development process of ontology translation system.

used. For each task of each activity we use the same structure: we describe the objectives of the task, the input and output, the participants, and the techniques recommended.

We will use examples to illustrate each of the tasks described. All these examples have been extracted from the WebODE export service to OWL DL.

Table 3.2. List of activities and tasks of the method for developing ontology translation systems.

Activity	***Task***
1. Feasibility study	1.1. Identify ontology translation system scope 1.2. Analyze current ontology translation systems 1.3. Define ontology translation system requirements 1.4. Decide about the feasibility of the system
2. Analysis of source and target formats	2.1. Describe source and target formats 2.2. Determine expressiveness of source and target formats 2.3. Compare knowledge models of source and target formats 2.4. Describe and compare additional features of source and target formats 2.5. Determine the scope of translation decisions 2.6. Specify test plan
3. Design of the translation system	3.1. Find and reuse similar translation systems 3.2. Propose transformations at the pragmatic level 3.3. Propose transformations at the semantic level 3.4. Propose transformations at the syntax level 3.5. Propose transformations at the lexical level 3.6. Propose additional transformations
4. Implementation of the translation system	4.1. Find translation functions to be reused 4.2. Implement transformations in the pragmatic level 4.3. Implement transformations in the semantic level 4.4. Implement transformations in the syntax level 4.5. Implement transformations in the lexical level 4.6. Implement additional transformations 4.7. Process declarative specification and integrate the system 4.8. Execute test suite

3.4.1 Activity 1. Feasibility Study

In software engineering, the objective of the feasibility study is to analyze the idea or need for a software system, potential approaches, and all its life cycle constraints and benefits [IEEE Standard 1074-1995, 1996]. The feasibility study may consider modeling and prototyping techniques and may suggest whether to make or buy the system, partially or totally. Besides, each recommendation must be fully justified, documented and formally approved by all concerned organizations (including the user and the developer).

In our specific case, the objective of this activity is to analyze the current ontology translation needs of the organization so that the proposed solution takes into account not only the technical restrictions (technical feasibility), but also other restrictions related to the business objectives of the organization (business feasibility) and to the project actions that can be successfully undertaken (project feasibility). As a result of this activity, the main requisites to be satisfied by the ontology translation system are obtained, and the main costs, benefits, and risks are identified. The most important aspect of this feasibility study concerns the technical restrictions, which can determine whether it is recommended or not to continue with the ontology translation system development.

Our proposal for organizing this activity into tasks is inspired by the tasks proposed by [METRICA v.3] for the feasibility study process of software systems; however, the techniques (and documents) used in the execution of these tasks are inspired by knowledge engineering approaches (such as [Gómez-Pérez et al., 1997] and [Schreiber et al., 1999]).

As shown in figure 3.6, we first propose determining the scope of the ontology translation system to be implemented, the expected outcome of such a system, the context in which it will be used, etc. We then propose analyzing the current translation systems available, if any, and determining the requisites to be accomplished by the new system. Finally, we propose filling in a checklist where the three dimensions identified above are considered (technical, business, and project feasibility) to allow making a decision on the feasibility of the system and to propose a set of actions and recommendations to be followed.

Consequently, the input to this activity consists in some preliminary high-level information about the current system, the knowledge representation and reasoning (KRR) needs, and the source and target formats. The results consist in a deeper description of the current ontology translation systems available for the origin and target formats, a preliminary catalogue of requisites for the system to be developed, and the recommendation about its feasibility including the main costs, benefits, and risks involved.

A summary of the results obtained, techniques used, and participants of each task is presented in table 3.3. In the rest of this section we will describe in detail each of the tasks within this activity.

Task 1.1. Identify Ontology Translation System Scope

In this task we must determine the scope of the ontology translation system with the aim of providing a high-level description of the translation system needed. This high-level description will mainly address the expected outcome of the translation system, the context where it will be used, the ontology components to which it will be applied, etc.

To perform this task, all the people involved in the project will participate, including the knowledge and software engineers, the project manager and the executive manager. The techniques to be used are mainly interviews with the executive manager and joint brainstorming sessions where the main requisites of such a system are to be determined.

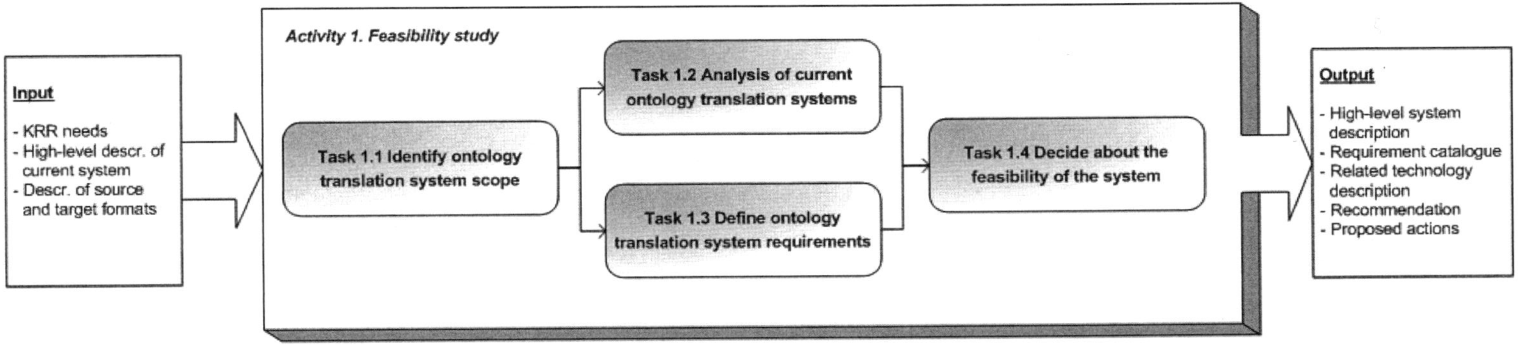

Figure 3.6. Task decomposition of activity 1 (feasibility study).

Task	*Products*	*Techniques*	*Participants*
Task 1.1. Identify ontology translation system scope	High-level system description	Interviews Brainstorming	Project manager Knowledge engineer Software engineer
Task 1.2. Analyse current ontology translation systems	High-level description of related translation technology	Interviews Cataloguing	Project manager Knowledge engineer Software engineer Expert users
Task 1.3. Define ontology translation system requirements	Requirement catalogue	Cataloguing	Project manager Knowledge engineer Software engineer Expert users
Task 1.4. Decide about the feasibility of the system	Recommendation Proposed actions	Checklists	Executive manager Project manager Knowledge engineer Software engineer

Table 3.3. Task products, techniques and participants of activity 1 (feasibility study).

Input products and output results

Input: knowledge representation and reasoning needs in the target format.

Output: high-level system description.

Participants

Project manager, knowledge engineers, and software engineers.

Techniques

Interviews and brainstorming sessions.

Practical example

Let us assume that we have to develop an ontology translation system from the WebODE platform to OWL. The reason for developing such a system is that we want to make WebODE ontologies available in that language, since we consider that it will be widely used in the future as a standard for developing ontologies for the Semantic Web.

After several interviews with people who have developed ontologies in OWL, and after several brainstorming sessions held up with the members of the Ontological Engineering group at UPM, we have come up with a high-level description of the translation system to be developed:

"The WebODE ontology export service to OWL will perform ontology translations to the OWL DL sublanguage. It will not export ontologies to OWL Lite since this sublanguage is too restrictive and much knowledge would be lost in the translation process, nor will it export ontologies to OWL Full, since we want to have decidable inference systems for the ontologies generated.

The export service has to be integrated in the WebODE platform. It will not be developed as a backend, because we do not care about maintaining knowledge in cyclic transformations to and from OWL; that requisite could be considered in the future. We just want to be able to export WebODE ontologies to that language so as to make them available for their use in the Semantic Web. Therefore, the system to be developed will be available as an export service that any WebODE user can use at any time during the ontology development process, even though it will be normally used once that the ontology is finished.

The WebODE export service to OWL DL will be widely used in the future, and we consider its development as a strategic part of the WebODE workbench and as a contribution to the Semantic Web vision.

Finally, we should take into account that the OWL DL specification has been recently proposed as a W3C Recommendation (February 2004). It may have modifications in the short, medium and long term."

Task 1.2. Analyze Current Ontology Translation Systems

The goal of this task is to analyze existing ontology translation systems that can be reused, either partially or totally, for the new development. The ontology translation systems to be analyzed include translation systems between the source and target formats, between earlier versions of the source and/or target formats, between the source format and other similar target formats, etc. It may also include the analysis of indirect transformations, that is, transformations from the source to the target by means of other intermediate formats.

Among the participants in this task we may include expert users of the source and target formats, if available. Expert users may provide indicators to analyze whether the target format is similar to another for which there is currently support (hence its translation system could be reused). Experts can also provide information about which expressions are more widely used than others in the source and target formats.

Regarding the techniques to be used to achieve this task, we mainly recommend performing interviews with expert users and applying cataloguing practices to collect the details of the related translation technology.

Input products and output results

Input: high-level descriptions of the system to be developed, of the current translation systems, and of the source and target formats.

Output: catalogue of the related translation technology and recommendations for reuse.

Participants

Project manager, knowledge and software engineers, and expert users.

Techniques

Interviews and cataloguing.

Practical example

Following the previous example, we analyze the ontology translation systems that could be reused when developing our WebODE export service to OWL DL. In a first step, and after an interview with experts in ontology markup languages, we select the WebODE export services to RDF(S), OIL and DAML+OIL, the DAML+OIL to OWL converter, the OWL plug-in for Protégé-2000, and the Jena2 library.

After analyzing these systems, we obtain the following conclusions:

"1. We can reuse the WebODE export service to RDF(S), because OWL DL instances are expressed in RDF.

2. We can also reuse some parts of the WebODE export service to DAML+OIL, since DAML+OIL and OWL are similar to each other.

3. OIL is also similar to OWL. However, the current WebODE export service to OIL generates the output in a plain text format, which is not reusable for our objective, and many of the most complex translation decisions are already considered in the DAML+OIL export service.

4. The DAML+OIL to OWL converter does not work properly in some cases, generating non valid OWL files. Besides, this would require making two transformations (from WebODE to DAML+OIL first, and then from DAML+OIL to OWL), which would make the system hardly efficient for large ontologies.

5. The OWL plug-in is too specific for Protégé-2000 ontologies, and has been implemented as a backend, with a strong interaction with the Protégé-2000 ontology management API. Hence it cannot be easily reused.

6. The Jena2 library provides an easy-to-use Java API to generate OWL ontologies in any of its allowed formats (RDF/XML, RDF/XML Abbrev, N3, etc.)."

From the above conclusions the catalogue of translation systems that should be considered for partial or total reuse is the following:

"- *WebODE export service to RDF(S)*. RDF export can be reused in OWL instance generation. The service is already integrated in WebODE and has been developed with this method.

- *WebODE export service to DAML+OIL*. Several translation decisions can be reused since DAML+OIL is based on description logics, as OWL DL.

- *Jena2 library*. It provides an easy-to-use Java API to generate OWL files automatically."

Task 1.3. Define Ontology Translation System Requirements

In this task we define the catalogue of high-level requirements of the ontology translation system. This catalogue considers both the functional requirements (the ontology components to be transformed, the expected outcomes regarding knowledge preservation and pragmatic preservation, etc.) and the non-functional requirements (aspects related to the integration with other systems, the expected performance of the translation system, the context where it will be used, etc.).

This task is performed in parallel to the task 1.2, and by the same participants, with interviews to elicit the requirements, and cataloguing practices to document them.

Input products and output results

Input: high-level descriptions of the system and of the source and target formats.

Output: catalogue of requirements of the ontology translation system.

Participants

Project manager, knowledge and software engineers, and expert users.

Techniques

Interviews and cataloguing.

Practical example

In our example, the following requirements are elicited:

"***Functional requirements***:

Req1. The ontology translation system does not aim at preserving all the knowledge represented in the ontology, but only those pieces of knowledge that can be directly transformed into OWL DL, without workarounds. Regarding pragmatics, the transformations to be made must ensure that the resulting OWL DL ontologies are easy to understand for OWL-aware human users and systems.

Req2. The WebODE knowledge model components to be translated to OWL DL are the following: concepts and their instance attributes, ad hoc relations, concept taxonomies (including subclass-of relationships, disjoint and exhaustive concept decompositions, and concept partitions), and instances.

Req3. The WebODE knowledge model component to be translated partially to OWL DL is the following: formal axioms that can be transformed to OWL DL.

Req4. The WebODE knowledge model components that will not be translated to OWL DL are the following: class attributes, synonyms and acronyms, bibliographic references, and rules.

Req5. WebODE attribute datatypes will be transformed into XML Schema datatypes.

Req6. WebODE instance sets will be transformed into separate RDF files.

Non-functional requirements:

Req7. The translation system must be integrated in the WebODE platform as an export service, providing the user with a ZIP file that contains the OWL DL ontology file and the instances' files.

Req8. There are no specific requirements related to the performance of the transformations to be made by the WebODE export service to OWL DL."

Task 1.4. Decide about the Feasibility of the System

The objective of this task is to make a decision on the feasibility of the ontology translation system to be developed, and to recommend which specific actions should be taken into account to overcome the problems that may arise during its development.

In this task, all the key implications obtained in the previous tasks are wrapped up to support the decision-making process. They are summarized in a checklist, inspired by the worksheet OM-5 proposed by the CommonKADS methodology [Schreiber et al., 1999] and adapted to the specific development of ontology translation systems. In this checklist we stress more the technical feasibility than the other two (business and project feasibility).

If the project is considered feasible, the proposed actions (included in the questionnaire presented below) help to prepare the beginning of the translation system development and are the main input of the subsequent activities. These actions determine the number of iterations in the development process and the ontology components transformed in each iteration. In addition, the main costs, benefits, and risks of the development are identified.

Input products and output results

Input: catalogue of requirements of the ontology translation system, catalogue of the related translated technology and recommendations for reuse; high-level descriptions of the system to be developed, of the current translation systems, and of the source and target formats, and knowledge representation and reasoning needs in the target format.

Output: recommendations and proposed actions

Participants

Executive manager, project manager, knowledge engineers, and software engineers.

Techniques

Usage of checklists. We recommend to use a checklist based on the CommonKADS feasibility decision making worksheet (OM-5). This checklist is presented in table 3.4.

The questions that appear in it should not be considered exhaustive: users may add as many questions and answers as they want to help in the decision-making process.

Table 3.4. Checklist for the feasibility decision making (based on the CommonKADS worksheet OM-5 [Schreiber et al., 1999]).

	Checklist for feasibility decision making
Business feasibility	1. What are the expected benefits for the organization from the development of an ontology translation system? 2. How large is the expected value? 3. Will the ontology translation system be used for a long-term period? 4. What are the expected costs for the ontology translation system development? 5. How does this compare to possible alternative solutions, such as performing translations by hand or by means of intermediate translation systems?
Project feasibility	1. Is there adequate commitment from the actors and stakeholders involved? 2. Can the resources needed in terms of time, budget, equipment, and staffing be made available? 3. Are the required knowledge and other competencies available? 4. Are the expectations regarding the project and its results realistic? 5. Are the project organization and its internal and external communication adequate? 6. Are there further project risks and uncertainties?
Technical feasibility	With regard to the source format: 1. Do the project participants have a deep knowledge of the source format (including the knowledge model components and the reasoning services available)? 2. Does the source format have a clear and well-defined Java API? 3. Have the project participants built and/or used ontologies in the source format? With regard to the target format: 4. Do the project participants have a deep knowledge of the target format (including the knowledge model components and the reasoning services available)? 5. Does the target format have a clear and well-defined Java API? 6. Have the project participants built and/or used ontologies in the target format? With regard to the transformation process: 7. Are the source and target formats based on the same KR paradigms? 8. Does the ontology translation system need to translate the ontology completely or partially? 9. Does the ontology translation system need to preserve all the knowledge in the transformation? 10. Does the ontology translation system need to preserve completely the pragmatics of the ontology in the transformation? 11. Is it clear what the success measures are and how to test the validity, quality, and satisfactory performance? 12. How complex, in terms of knowledge stored and reasoning processes to be carried out, is the translation process? With regard to the non-functional requirements: 13. How complex is the interaction with other information systems and possible other resources? Are state-of-the-art methods and techniques available and adequate? 14. Are there any specific requirements about the ontology translation system performance? 15. Are there critical aspects involved, relating to time, quality, needed resources, or otherwise? 16. Are there further technological risks and uncertainties?
Proposed actions	1. Focus: What is the recommended focus on the problem-opportunity areas? 2. Target solution: What is the recommended solution direction for this focus area? 3. What are the expected results, costs, and benefits? 4. What project actions are required to get there? 5. How many development iterations will be performed, and which components will be transformed in each iteration? 6. Risks: If circumstances inside or outside the organization change, under which conditions is it wise to reconsider the proposed decisions?

Practical example

In our example, we filled the checklist and obtained the result presented in table 3.5:

Table 3.5. Checklist for the feasibility decision making of the WebODE export service to OWL DL

	Checklist for feasibility decision making
Business feasibility	The organization expects large benefits from the development of the WebODE export service to OWL DL, because WebODE will be one of the first ontology platforms with OWL support. We expect that the WebODE user community will grow. The export service will be used for a long-term period. It may require slight modifications during its life, due to the recent proposal of the OWL language to W3C Recommendation. The expected cost of developing such a service is around 2 man-month. The other alternatives explored (transforming OWL ontologies through DAML+OIL or through other ontology tools) have several drawbacks: we are dependent on their support for new updates of the OWL specification, and they would have a negative impact on the performance of the translation system.
Project feasibility	People in the organization are committed to the development of the WebODE export service to OWL DL, and all the resources needed will be made available. The developers of the translation service have experience in the development of other translation systems with the same method, and have also a deep knowledge of the main features of the knowledge models of WebODE and OWL DL. The expectations are realistic, and the communication channels between the people involved are adequate. The development team has good communication with the OWL developers. The only risks foreseen are those related to the changes that the OWL language specifications may suffer. However, the language has been already published as a W3C Recommendation, and we only foresee minor changes.
Technical feasibility	***With regard to the source format:*** The project participants have a deep and sound knowledge of the source format (WebODE) and of its Java API. They have also built and used a large number of WebODE ontologies. ***With regard to the target format:*** The project participants have a good knowledge of the target format (OWL DL) and of the Jena2 library, which will be used as its API. They have also built and used some OWL ontologies. ***With regard to the transformation process:*** WebODE and OWL DL are based on different KR paradigms: a combination of frames and first order logic and description logic, respectively. The ontology must be translated almost completely to OWL DL, since we want to lose as less knowledge as possible in the transformation process. We do not aim at preserving all the knowledge of the ontology, but we do at preserving the pragmatics of what we transform. Several test ontologies will be defined to test for the satisfactory performance of the export service developed. Transforming the frames KR paradigm into description logic is a complex task that requires implementing difficult translation decisions: such as transforming the scope of ad hoc relations and instance attributes from being local to concepts to being global to the ontology, transforming concept and instance attribute definitions into property restrictions, etc. However, there are already similar translation systems implemented that may help to make these translation decisions. ***With regard to the non-functional requirements:*** The interaction with WebODE is complex though well known by the project participants, and the interaction with the Jena2 library is considered easy to carry out. No specific requirements about the system performance exist not critical aspects or risks about time, quality, needed resources, etc.
Proposed actions	Our recommendation is to create the WebODE export service to OWL DL reusing the Jena2 library and part of the WebODE export service to RDF(S). We will also reuse some of the translation decisions performed for the WebODE export service to DAML+OIL. We foresee great benefits from the development of this system, which will increase the WebODE user community and will allow developing ontologies for the Semantic Web with its ontology editor. The development of the export service will be performed in three iterations: first, the WebODE concepts, attributes, ad hoc relations, simple concept taxonomies, and instances will be transformed; then, we will deal with complex primitives for creating concept taxonomies, such as disjoint and exhaustive decompositions, and partitions; finally, we will deal with WebODE formal axioms and will perform all the pragmatic transformations. The only risks foreseen are related to the fact that the OWL language has been published as a W3C Recommendation very recently, and consequently may suffer from minor changes in the near future.

3.4.2 Activity 2. Analysis of Source and Target Formats

The objective of this activity is to obtain a thorough description and comparison of the source and target formats of the ontology translation system. We assume that this comparison will allow gaining a better understanding of their similarities and differences in expressiveness, which will be useful to design and implement the translation decisions in the subsequent activities. Besides, in this activity we will refine the catalogue of requirements already obtained as a result of the feasibility study, and we will identify the test suite to be used to test the translation system validity after each iteration in its development process.

To perform the description and comparison tasks we can use formal, semi-formal or informal approaches, which are identified in chapter 1. As we will see, we recommend the semi-formal and informal approaches, which are more informative and useful for the specific task of developing ontology translation systems. However, this fact does not prevent us from using any of the formal approaches that have been proposed so far in the literature, and which could help us to determine formally whether an expression of the source format can be transformed into the target format without losses of knowledge.

Once the two formats have been described, evaluated, and compared, we recommend focusing on other additional features that could be needed in the translation process. These may include reasoning mechanisms or any other specific details that could be interesting for the translation task. For these description and comparison tasks we can follow formal, semi-formal or informal approaches. Again, we recommend the semi-formal and informal ones.

The information gathered in the preceding tasks is used to determine the scope of the translation decisions to be made: which components map to each other, which components of the source format must be represented by means of others in the target format, which components cannot be represented in the target format, etc. As a result, we get a refinement of the catalogue of requirements obtained during the feasibility study, which serves as the basis for the next activities (design and implementation of the translation system).

Finally, we propose defining the test plan, which consists of a set of unitary tests that the translation system must pass in order to be considered valid. We will define a test suite consisting of several ontologies covering all the possible translation situations that the translation system must cover. These ontologies should be available in the source format and in the target format (which is the output of the translation process). The test execution will consist on comparing the output obtained and the output expected. For each iteration of the software development process we will define different sets of ontologies.

Consequently, this activity receives as an input all the results of the feasibility study together with the description of the source and target formats –which was also used as an input for that activity– and outputs a comparison of both formats, the scope of the translation decisions to be performed with a refined requirements catalogue, and a test plan with its corresponding test suite.

This activity is mainly performed by the knowledge engineer that will be in charge of designing and implementing the translation decisions, with the help of expert users that determine the expressiveness of the source and target formats, and of software engineers that describe additional features of the formats, determine the scope of translation decisions, and specify the test plan. The project manager will help in the refinement of the requirements catalogue.

A summary of the tasks to be performed in this activity and their timeline is presented in figure 3.7. The results obtained, techniques used and participants of each task are summarized in table 3.6.

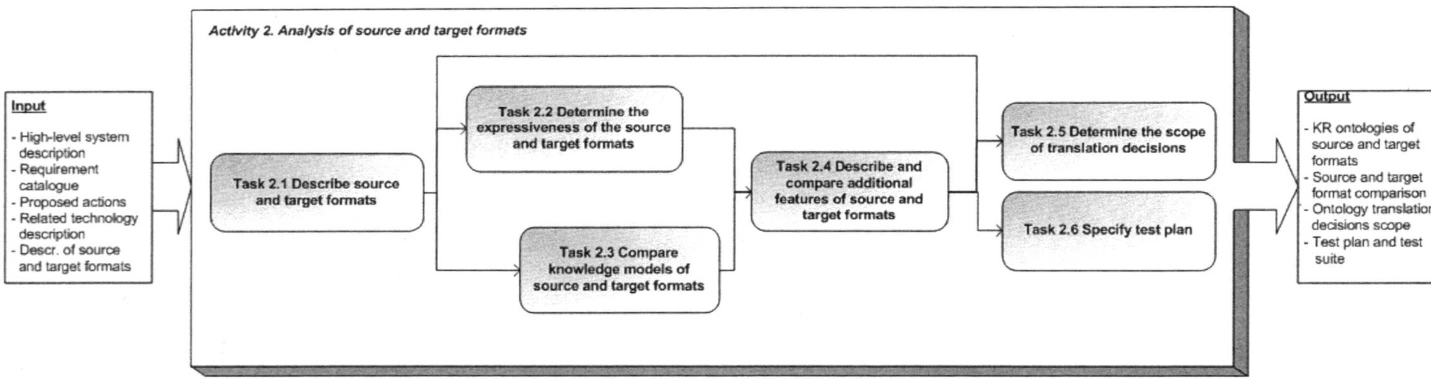

Figure 3.7. Task decomposition of activity 2 (analysis of source and target formats).

Task	*Products*	*Techniques*	*Participants*
Task 2.1. Describe source and target formats	KR ontologies of source and target formats	KR ontologies	Knowledge engineer
Task 2.2. Determine expressiveness of source and target formats	Evaluation of expressiveness of source and target formats	Formal semantics Informal evaluation approaches	Knowledge engineer Expert users
Task 2.3. Compare knowledge models of source and target formats	Comparison of source and target format knowledge models	Formal comparison approaches Venn diagrams Evaluation frameworks	Knowledge engineer
Task 2.4. Describe and compare additional features of source and target formats	Comparison of source and target format additional features	Cataloguing	Knowledge engineer Software engineer
Task 2.5. Determine scope of translation decisions	Scope of ontology translation decisions Refined requirement catalogue	Cataloguing	Project manager Knowledge engineer Software engineer
Task 2.6. Specify test plan	Test plan Test suite	System tests	Knowledge engineer Software engineer

Table 3.6. Task products, techniques and participants of activity 2 (analysis of source and target formats).

Task 2.1. Describe Source and Target Formats

In this task we provide a detailed description of the source and target formats by means of their knowledge representation ontologies (aka KR ontologies). The advantage of using KR ontologies is that they present the primitives to be used when building ontologies. Besides, the KR class taxonomy provides a hierarchy of some of those primitives. This description will be used as an input for other tasks inside this activity.

A knowledge engineer will be in charge of these detailed descriptions. He/she will analyze the documentation available for each format, focusing especially on their knowledge models and on the ontology components that they can represent.

Input products and output results

Input: documentation of source and target formats.

Output: KR ontologies of the source and target formats.

Participants

Knowledge engineer.

Techniques

KR ontology description, with its class taxonomies and its list of properties. These types of descriptions can be found in the documentation of ontology markup languages such as OIL [Horrocks et al., 2000]. They can be also found at [Gómez-Pérez et al., 2003] for the ontology markup languages RDF(S), DAML+OIL, and OWL.

Practical example

We show an extract of the description of the OWL DL language. A more complete description can be found in [Gómez-Pérez et al., 2003, pages 65-71]:

"The OWL language [Dean and Schreiber, 2004] was published as a W3C Recommendation in February 2004. It is derived from the DAML+OIL language, and it builds upon RDF(S). OWL is divided in layers: OWL Lite, OWL DL, and OWL Full. OWL Lite extends RDF(S) and gathers the most common features of OWL; therefore it is intended for users that only need to create class taxonomies and simple constraints. OWL DL includes the complete OWL vocabulary. OWL Full provides more flexibility than OWL DL to represent ontologies but it does not ensure that there will be decidable reasoners available for it.

OWL DL is based on the description logic language SHOIN(d+). The OWL DL KR ontology, which is implemented in OWL, is available at: *http://www.w3.org/2002/07/owl*. It has 40 primitives (16 classes and 24 properties). Figure 3.8 shows the class taxonomy of the primitives that are classes in the OWL KR ontology. All these primitives belong to OWL Lite. Hence, they also belong to OWL DL and OWL Full. These primitives can be grouped as follows:

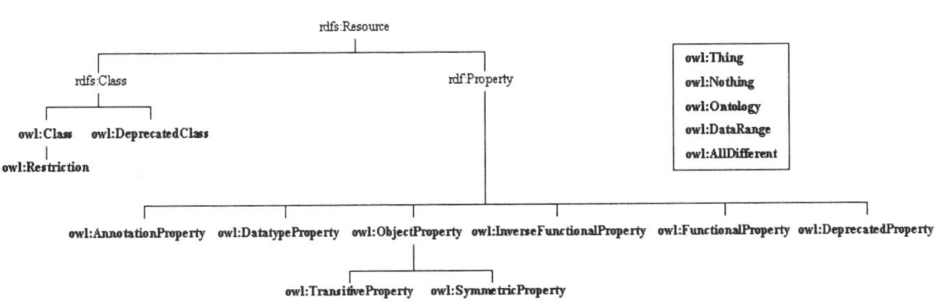

Figure 3.8. Class taxonomy of the OWL DL KR ontology.

- **Classes for defining classes and restrictions** (*owl:Class* and *owl:Restriction*). The primitive *owl:Class* specializes *rdfs:Class* and is used to define classes. The primitive *owl:Restriction* specializes *owl:Class* and is used to define property restrictions for classes (number restrictions, existential restrictions, universal restrictions, etc.).

[...]

OWL class expressions are built with KR primitives that are properties. Some of them belong to OWL Lite and others belong to OWL DL. Table 3.7 summarizes the main features of the properties of the OWL KR ontology, specifying their domain and range. If the value for the range is "not specified", we mean that the property can take any value which is not restricted to a specific class of the OWL KR ontology. Besides, in OWL we can use the properties *rdfs:subClassOf*, *rdfs:subPropertyOf*, *rdfs:domain*, *rdfs:range*, *rdfs:comment*, *rdfs:label*, *rdfs:seeAlso*, and *rdfs:isDefinedBy* from the RDF(S) KR ontology.

Table 3.7. Property descriptions of the OWL DL KR ontology.

Property name	domain	range
owl:intersectionOf	owl:Class	rdf:List
owl:unionOf	owl:Class	rdf:List
owl:complementOf	owl:Class	owl:Class
owl:oneOf	owl:Class	rdf:List
owl:onProperty	owl:Restriction	rdf:Property
owl:allValuesFrom	owl:Restriction	rdfs:Class
owl:hasValue	owl:Restriction	*not specified*
owl:someValuesFrom	owl:Restriction	rdfs:Class
owl:minCardinality	owl:Restriction	xsd:nonNegativeInteger
owl:maxCardinality	owl:Restriction	xsd:nonNegativeInteger
owl:cardinality	owl:Restriction	xsd:nonNegativeInteger
owl:inverseOf	owl:ObjectProperty	owl:ObjectProperty
owl:sameAs	owl:Thing	owl:Thing
owl:equivalentClass	owl:Class	owl:Class
owl:equivalentProperty	rdf:Property	rdf:Property
owl:sameIndividualAs	owl:Thing	owl:Thing
owl:differentFrom	owl:Thing	owl:Thing
owl:disjointWith	owl:Class	owl:Class
owl:distinctMembers	owl:AllDifferent	rdf:List
owl:versionInfo	*not specified*	*not specified*
owl:priorVersion	owl:Ontology	owl:Ontology
owl:incompatibleWith	owl:Ontology	owl:Ontology
owl:backwardCompatibleWith	owl:Ontology	owl:Ontology
owl:imports	owl:Ontology	owl:Ontology

The OWL KR primitives can be grouped as follows:

- **Properties for defining class expressions**:
    - Class conjunction (*owl:intersectionOf*), disjunction (*owl:unionOf*), and negation (*owl:complementOf*).
    - Property restrictions. They are defined with the class *owl:Restriction*. Restrictions are defined with two elements: *owl:onProperty* (which refers to the property name) and another element that expresses value restriction (*owl:allValuesFrom*), existential restriction (*owl:someValuesFrom*), and number restriction (*owl:cardinality*, *owl:maxCardinality*, and *owl:minCardinality*).

[...]"

Task 2.2. Determine Expressiveness of Source and Target Formats

This task aims at determining clearly the expressiveness of each of the formats involved in the transformation. To achieve this objective, we can use different kinds of techniques, based on formal, semi-formal, and informal approaches:

- Formal techniques have been widely used to describe the semantics of KR systems. They are known as model-theoretic semantics because they use model theories[31] [Manzano, 1999] to determine the semantics. Other formal techniques consist in defining mappings between the format whose semantics is described to another format with a well-defined model-theoretic semantics.
- Semi-formal techniques determine which knowledge model components can be defined in a format. They usually consist of evaluation frameworks that provide checklists with details of all the knowledge model components that can be represented in KR systems.

[31] *Among the many bibliographic references that could be used to refer to model theory, one of the basic textbooks has been selected.*

- Informal techniques also determine which knowledge model components can be defined in a format, but without using specific evaluation frameworks nor checklists. They usually consist in enumerating the knowledge model components that can be defined in each KR format.

Given that our aim is to develop ontology translation systems between different formats, we recommend using the semi-formal and informal approaches because they provide coarse-grained overviews of the components that can be defined in each format.

This task is performed by the same knowledge engineer, with the help of experts in the source and target formats. Once the expressiveness of both formats has been defined, we will be able to compare them and propose the translations to be implemented by the ontology translation system.

Input products and output results

Input: detailed description of source and target formats.

Output: formal, semi-formal or informal semantics of the source and target formats.

Participants

Knowledge engineer and expert users.

Techniques

Formal approaches to define semantics: model theory and mappings to other formats.

Semi-formal approaches to define semantics: evaluation frameworks [Corcho and Gómez-Pérez, 2000].

Informal approaches to define semantics: unstructured enumerations and informal descriptions of knowledge components [Garshol, 2001; Garshol, 2003; Gil and Ratnakar, 2002; Noy et al., 2001].

Practical example

Table 3.8 shows the results of applying the evaluation framework described in [Corcho and Gómez-Pérez, 2000] to the source and target formats of the ontology translation system to be developed: WebODE and OWL DL respectively. The cells in the table are filled with the symbol '+' to indicate that it is a supported feature in the format, '-' for non supported features, and 'W' for non supported features that could be supported with some workaround.

Table 3.8. Results of applying the evaluation framework described in [Corcho and Gómez-Pérez, 2000] to the knowledge models of WebODE and OWL DL.

	WebODE	OWL DL
CONCEPTS	+	+
Metaclasses	+	-
Attributes		
Instance attributes	+	+
Class attributes	+	-
Facets		
Type constraints	+	+
Cardinality constraints	+	+
Procedural knowledge	-	-
CONCEPT TAXONOMIES		
Subclass-Of	+	+
Disjoint-Decomposition	+	+
Exhaustive-Decomposition	+	W
Partition	+	W

	WebODE	OWL DL
RELATIONS		
Binary relations	+	+
n-ary relations	W	W
Relation hierarchies	W	+
Integrity constraints	-	-
OTHER		
Formal Axioms	+	-
Instances	+	+
Rules	+	-

An informal description of the WebODE knowledge model semantics can be found at [Corcho et al., 2002], and several formal semantics for OWL DL can be found at [Patel-Schneider et al., 2004].

Task 2.3. Compare Knowledge Models of Source and Target Formats

The objective of this task is to provide a comprehensive comparison of the knowledge models of the source and target formats. This comparison and the detailed description obtained in task 2.2 are used to propose the translations to be performed between the formats. This task is accomplished by the knowledge engineer, who has to decide which components are equivalent though they may be named differently, which details differ, etc.

The format of the results obtained from this task is determined by the kind of technique used to carry out the comparison. As in task 2.2, we can use formal, semi-formal, and informal techniques. Here we also recommend the semi-formal and informal techniques, because they are more informative and useful for developing ontology translation systems.

Input products and output results

Input: detailed description of the source and target formats.

Output: comparison of the source and target formats.

Participants

Knowledge engineer.

Techniques

Formal comparisons ([Baader, 1996], [Borgida, 1996], [Euzenat and Stuckenschmidt, 2002], etc.). They are based on the definition of formal semantics described in section 1.3.

Informal and semi-formal comparisons, based on evaluation frameworks [Corcho and Gómez-Pérez, 2000], Venn diagrams [Knublauch, 2003] or tables describing how different ontology components are represented in each language [Garshol, 2001; Garshol, 2003; Gil and Ratnakar, 2002; Noy et al., 2001].

Practical example

The results presented in table 3.8 permit determining the main aspects to be considered when translating from WebODE into OWL DL; these aspects are derived from the differences shown in the table. Some of these differences are due to the fact that the WebODE knowledge model is based on a combination of frames and first order logic, while the OWL DL knowledge model is based on description logics:

- Class attributes cannot be represented in OWL DL. This type of attributes is useful to describe characteristics of the classes that are not inherited by their subclasses nor by their instances.
- In OWL DL there are not specific primitives for representing exhaustive decompositions of classes (and consequently, nor are there primitives for partitions). This kind of knowledge must be expressed by stating that the superclass is equivalent to the union of all the classes in the decomposition or partition, and that all these classes are subclasses of the superclass.
- N-ary relations between classes must be represented similarly in both formats: by creating a class that simulates the relation.
- WebODE represents relation hierarchies by means of formal axioms, while OWL DL represents them with a specific primitive (*rdfs:subPropertyOf*).
- WebODE allows representing any first order logic axiom and any rule. The formal axioms that can be represented in OWL DL are restricted and rules cannot be represented. This fact will be considered in the future in another language that will be built on top of OWL (e.g., OWL Rule, SWRL).

This preliminary list does not pretend to be exhaustive but to provide some guidance for the analysis of the main sources of differences that will be relevant for the translation."

Task 2.4. Describe and Compare Additional Features of Source and Target Formats

In this task we describe and compare those features of the source and target formats that are not considered by the previous knowledge model descriptions and comparisons, and that the knowledge and software engineers may consider interesting from the point of view of ontology translation. For instance, the source and target formats may have different reasoning mechanisms attached, may require different parameters for representing the ontologies (namespaces, documentation options, etc.), may provide different visualization options for the ontologies (in the case of ontology tools), etc.

Input products and output results

Input: detailed description of the source and target format knowledge models and evaluation of expressiveness and comparison of source and target formats.

Output: catalogue of the similarities and differences between the source and target formats that are not specifically related to their knowledge models or that are not covered by the informal, semi-formal, and formal comparison approaches described previously.

Participants

Knowledge and software engineers.

Techniques

Cataloguing.

Practical example

Besides the differences between the WebODE and OWL DL knowledge models, obtained as a result of the preceding tasks, we also have the following:

- WebODE ontologies can contain bibliographic references, which can be associated to any ontology component.
- WebODE instance attributes contain more information than their correspondent components in OWL DL (datatype properties). In case of numeric attributes, they contain their minimum and maximum value, their measurement unit, and their precision. In addition, their datatypes are not restricted to a fixed set of built-in XML Schema datatypes, but any derived XML Schema datatype can be also used.
- The scope of the identifiers of WebODE instance attributes and ad hoc relations is local to the concept where they are defined (that is, their domain), while the scope of these identifiers in OWL DL is global to the ontology.
- Class definitions in OWL DL can be complete (expressing necessary and sufficient conditions to belong to the class) or partial (expressing only necessary conditions). Concept definitions are partial in WebODE. To express sufficient conditions in WebODE formal axioms must be used.
- OWL DL allows expressing unions of classes. These are expressed by means of formal axioms in WebODE.
- The WebODE reasoning engine implements attribute and relation inheritance, which is a typical functionality in frame-based systems. The available OWL DL reasoners mainly aim at detecting inconsistencies in class taxonomies, obtaining class subsumption relationships from class definitions, and some of them aim at detecting inconsistencies in instances.

Task 2.5. Determine the Scope of Translation Decisions

The objective of this task is to determine which components and expressions of the source format will be transformed into the target one, and which approaches will be taken to preserve the knowledge and the intended meaning of the ontology.

As we will see in chapter 4, the translation decisions to be taken can be driven by knowledge preservation constraints, by pragmatics preservation constraints, or by both at the same time, with different degrees of semantic and pragmatic preservation.

This task is performed jointly by the project manager and by the knowledge and software engineers, since many factors influence on the decisions to be proposed. As a result of this task, a refined catalogue of requirements for the ontology translation system will be output, where the transformations to be performed are more detailed than in the catalogue obtained during the feasibility study.

Input products and output results

Input: detailed description of the source and target format knowledge models, evaluation of expressiveness and comparison of source and target formats, and catalogue of additional similarities and differences between the source and target formats.

Output: scope of the ontology translation decisions and refined catalogue of requirements.

Participants

Project manager, and knowledge and software engineers.

Techniques

Cataloguing.

Practical example

The requisite catalogue obtained as a result of task 1.3 is refined, as shown below:

"***Functional requirements***:

Req1. The ontology translation system does not aim at preserving all the knowledge represented in the ontology, but only those pieces of knowledge that can be directly transformed to OWL DL, without workarounds, except for exhaustive concept decompositions and concept partitions. Regarding pragmatics, the transformations to be made must ensure that the resulting OWL DL ontologies are easy to understand for OWL-aware human users and systems.

Req2. The WebODE knowledge model components to be translated into OWL DL are the following: concepts and their instance attributes, ad hoc relations, concept taxonomies (including subclass-of relationships, disjoint and exhaustive concept decompositions, and concept partitions), and instances. The correspondences between these WebODE components and OWL DL components are shown in table 3.9:

Table 3.9. Correspondences between WebODE and OWL DL components.

WebODE component	OWL DL component
Concept	Class
Instance attribute (local scope)	Datatype property (global scope)
Ad hoc relation (local scope)	Object property (global scope)
Subclass of	Subclass of
Disjoint decompositions	Disjointness between pairs of classes
Exhaustive decompositions	Class equivalence to union of subclasses Subclass-of relationships
Partitions	Disjointness between pairs of classes Class equivalence to union of subclasses Subclass-of relationships
Instances	Individuals

Req3. The WebODE knowledge model component to be translated partially into OWL DL is the following: formal axioms that can be transformed into OWL DL.

Req4. The WebODE knowledge model components that will not be translated into OWL DL are the following: class attributes, synonyms and acronyms, bibliographic references, and rules.

Req5. WebODE attribute datatypes (including XML Schema datatypes) will be transformed into XML Schema datatypes. Derived XML Schema datatypes will be transformed into the XML Schema datatype *string*.

Req6. WebODE instance sets will be transformed to separate RDF files.

Non-functional requirements:

Req7. The translation system must be integrated in the WebODE platform as an export service, providing the user with a ZIP file that contains the OWL DL ontology file and the instances' files.

Req8. There are no specific requirements related to the performance of the transformations to be made by the WebODE export service to OWL DL."

Task 2.6. Specify Test Plan

This task, which is performed in parallel to the definition of the scope of ontology translation decisions, consists in defining the test plan for the ontology translation system.

As in general software development, in this phase we define the system tests to be used to test the validity of the generated ontology translation system.

The test suite consists of several ontologies that will cover all the possible translation situations the translation system must deal with. The ontologies are defined in the source and target formats, the latter being the expected output of the translation system when applied to the former. Consequently, each test execution will simply consist in comparing the output obtained when the translation system is applied to any of the source ontologies in the test suite with its corresponding target ontology.

Since the development of the translation system will be made iteratively, in each iteration we will define a new set of ontologies for the test suite, which must cover the ontologies used in the previous iteration plus new ontologies with the components being transformed in the current iteration.

This task is performed by the knowledge engineer, who decides which ontologies should be included in the test suite and generates manually their corresponding ontologies in the target format, and by the software engineer, who decides whether other aspects should be taken into account in the definition of these tests, such as input parameters for the ontology translation system, etc.

Input products and output results

Input: detailed description of the source and target format knowledge models, evaluation of expressiveness and comparison of source and target formats, and catalogue of additional similarities and differences between the source and target formats.

Output: ontology translation system test suite and test plan.

Participants

Knowledge and software engineers.

Techniques

System test cases.

Practical example

A subset of the synthetic ontologies described in [Corcho et al., 2003b] will be used as a test suite for the WebODE export service to OWL DL. This set of synthetic ontologies provides several combinations of those features that have to be tested to check the correct translation of ontologies by the ontology translation system developed (e.g., instance attributes with the same name defined for different concepts, with different types or with the same type, concepts and ad hoc relations with the same name, etc.).

For each of these WebODE ontologies, we have also defined the corresponding OWL ontology that is expected after the translation.

We are using synthetic ontologies because they allow combining all the possible translation situations considered by the ontology translation system. Besides, the test suite is divided in three groups, depending on the translations performed in each iteration of the ontology translation system development.

3.4.3 Activity 3. Design of the Translation System

The objective of the design activity is to provide a detailed specification of the transformations to be performed by the ontology translation system. From this specification we will obtain, in the implementation activity, the declarative implementation of the system, which will be used in its turn to generate the final ontology translation system.

As shown in figure 3.9, the tasks inside this activity are divided in three groups: a first group composed of only one task where similar ontology translation systems are analyzed for the sake of reuse, a second group composed of four tasks where the translation decisions in the four translation layers are proposed, and the last group composed of one task, where additional transformations, which do not fall in the previous translation layers, are proposed. We describe next the goals and responsible for each task, which are also summarized in table 3.10.

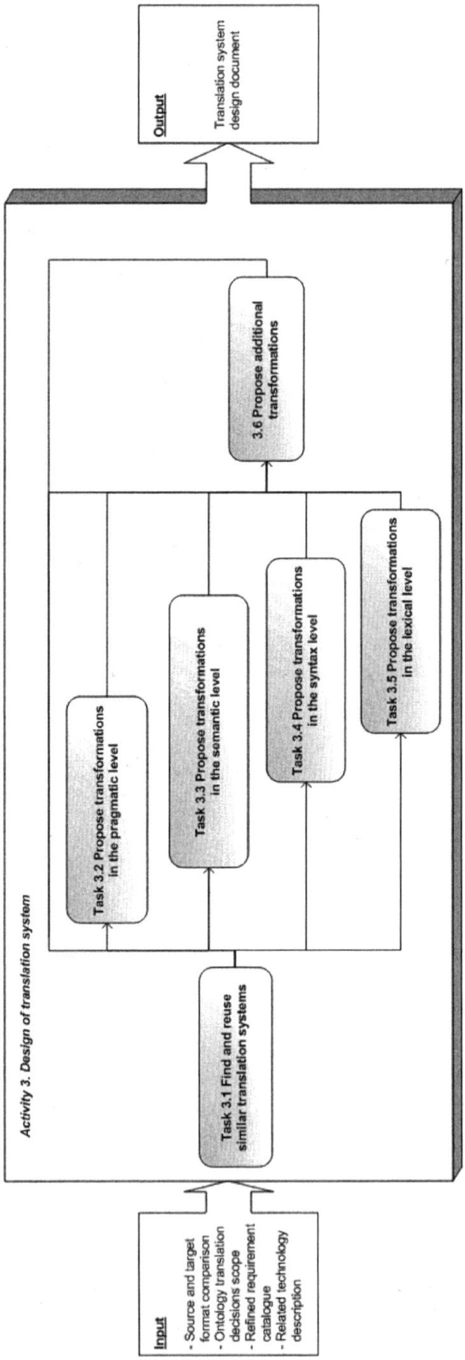

Figure 3.9. Task decomposition of activity 3 (design of the translation system).

Task	*Products*	*Techniques*	*Participants*
Task 3.1. Find and reuse similar translation systems	Catalogue of translation decisions to be reused	Cataloguing	Knowledge engineer Software engineer
Task 3.2. Propose transformations at the pragmatic level	Catalogue of translation decisions at the pragmatic level	Cataloguing Translation decision tables and diagrams	Knowledge engineer Software engineer
Task 3.3. Propose transformations at the semantic level	Catalogue of translation decisions at the semantic level	Cataloguing Translation decision tables and diagrams	Knowledge engineer Software engineer
Task 3.4. Propose transformations at the syntactic level	Catalogue of translation decisions at the syntax level	Cataloguing Translation decision tables and diagrams BNF grammar	Software engineer Knowledge engineer
Task 3.5. Propose transformations at the lexical level	Catalogue of translation decisions at the lexical level	Cataloguing Translation decision tables and diagrams BNF grammar	Software engineer Knowledge engineer
Task 3.6. Propose additional transformations	Catalogue of additional transformations	Cataloguing Translation decision tables Design patterns	Software engineer Knowledge engineer

Table 3.10. Task products, techniques and participants of activity 3 (design of the translation system).

The objective of the task in the first group is to analyze similar ontology translation systems and to detect which of their translation decisions can be actually reused. We assume that by reusing existing translation decisions we will be able to minimize the sources of errors in our translation proposals, and that we will be able to improve interoperability, since translation decisions are implemented similarly. Furthermore, we will benefit from work already known, of which we already know its properties (namely, how they preserve semantics and pragmatics). We must remember that the potential reusable systems were already identified and catalogued during the feasibility study. Therefore, the knowledge and software engineers will have to focus on those systems with two different purposes: the knowledge engineer will aim at detecting reusable translation decisions, while the software engineer will aim at detecting reusable pieces of software code.

The second group of tasks deals with the four layers of translation problems described in section 3.2: we propose to design transformations at the different inter-related levels, with different techniques for each layer, as we will describe later. All these tasks should be performed in parallel, and the decisions taken at one task provide feedback for the others, as shown in figure 3.9. We propose to use a top-down approach to design transformations: from the more abstract layer (pragmatic) to the most code-specific layer (lexical). As we presented elsewhere, translations will be driven by the pragmatic and semantic layers, and the decisions taken at the lower layers will be mainly influenced by the decisions taken in the more abstract ones.

The pragmatic and semantic translation decisions are typically made by knowledge engineers (it is recommended that these tasks are performed by the same persons that have carried out the analysis and comparison of the source and target formats). The syntax and lexical transformations can be proposed jointly by knowledge and software engineers, since they have more to do with general programming aspects rather than with the complexity of transforming knowledge. Besides, the software engineers can help in the pragmatic and semantic tasks by deciding whether the transformations that cannot be specified declaratively, due to its complexity, can be easily implemented in a general programming language or not.

Finally, the objective of the task in the last group is to propose any additional transformations or design issues not covered by the previous tasks, because they could not be catalogued as lexical, syntactic, semantic or pragmatic transformations, and which are necessary for the correct functioning of the ontology translation system. These transformations include design issues such as the initialization and setting up of parameters in the source and target formats, any integration needs foreseen of the generated system in the case of transformations where ontology tools or specific libraries are used, etc. This task will be mainly performed by software engineers, with the help of the knowledge engineers who have proposed the other types of transformations.

As shown in figure 3.9, we may need to come back to the second group of activities after proposing some additional transformations. This is a cyclic process that goes on until we determine all the transformations to be performed. All the output results obtained from the tasks in this activity are integrated in a single document called "translation system design document", as shown in the figure.

Task 3.1. Find and Reuse Similar Translation Systems

In this task we analyze the ontology translation systems selected during the feasibility study. Our objective is to detect parts of these translation systems that can be reused in ours, taking into account that now we have a better understanding of the differences between the source and target formats and of the software constraints.

Our assumption for proposing this task is that some translation decisions at all levels are normally reusable across different systems. We present two examples below:

- Let us suppose that the source format is a classical ontology language or an ontology tool with no support for the use of URIs, and that the target format is an ontology markup language. Hence the lexical transformations to be performed include transforming identifiers to valid URIs by using the appropriate XML encoding, removing invalid characters in URIs such as blank spaces, etc. The transformations to be performed will be similar no matter which the specific source and target formats are, provided that they belong to the previous groups.
- An interesting situation arises when the source and target formats belong to the same KR formalism than the source and target formats of another translation system available. In this case we will be able to reuse many translation decisions at the semantic and pragmatic levels. For example, let us suppose that we are transforming ontologies from a description-logic format to a frame-based format. Description logic formats allow defining concepts with complex expressions that may include the union and the negation of concepts. These complex expressions are not usually allowed in frame-based formats and normally we have to create anonymous classes to represent these expressions. The translation decisions are easily reusable if the source and target formats belong to those KR formalisms.

Similarly, we assume that many design decisions (e.g., those made for the sake of integrating the ontology translation system in an ontology tool or platform) can be reused, and hence the ontology translation system developers can also benefit from reusing those parts of the design of existing translation systems.

Consequently, in this task we will aim at reusing two types of elements: translation decisions, and software design decisions. The first subtask will be performed by knowledge engineers, while the second subtask will be performed by software engineers.

Input products and output results

Input: Related technology description, ontology translation decision scope, and refined requirement catalogue.

Output: Catalogue of translation decisions to be reused.

Participants

Knowledge and software engineers.

Techniques

Cataloguing

Practical example

As a result of the task 1.2 we determined the OWL API to be used and we obtained a catalogue of ontology translation systems that could be reused. The following specific aspects will be reused from each of them:

- *WebODE export service to RDF(S).*
  - o Translation decisions: each WebODE instance is transformed into an RDF resource, whose type is the class that corresponds to the WebODE concept of which the instance is instance of. The values for its instance attributes and for its ad hoc relations are also transformed to RDF.
  - o Software design decisions: for each WebODE instance set, this export service generates a file that contains the instances of the instance set. This is also the result expected for the WebODE export service to OWL DL, and hence it can be reused.
- *WebODE export service to DAML+OIL.*

- Translation decisions: OWL DL is based on a description logic similar to DAML+OIL's. Hence many translation decisions can be reused (e.g., those related to the transformation of the scope of instance attributes and ad hoc relations). We can also reuse the transformations of formal axioms to DAML+OIL expressions. However, there are other aspects that cannot be reused, such as the transformation of concept disjoint and exhaustive decompositions, and partitions, since in DAML+OIL they could be represented easily with specific primitives whilst in OWL DL a workaround must be done; or the transformations of instance attribute and ad hoc relation attachments into property restrictions because OWL DL does not define qualified property restrictions.
- Software design decisions: the file containing the ontology is output as a ZIP file in the WebODE export service to DAML+OIL. This is also the result expected for the WebODE export service to OWL DL, and therefore it can be reused.

Task 3.2. Propose Transformations at the Pragmatic Level

The objective of this task is to propose the set of transformations needed to comply with the restrictions related to the pragmatic preservation properties of the transformation. These restrictions were imposed during the analysis activity and described in the refined catalogue of requirements and in the ontology translation decision scope document.

This task will be performed by the knowledge engineers, who will describe in detail the transformations needed by means of diagrams and tables. This is the first task that we propose to start with, from the four-task group concerning transformations in the different translation layers, as shown in figure 3.9.

As described in section 3.2.4, the translation decisions taken at the pragmatic layer mainly consist in deciding which transformations to use when several can be used indistinctly. This is usually the case when it is possible to use different syntaxes or workarounds to express the same piece of knowledge, when we have different choices for the transformations of identifiers, etc. In this layer we also decide which components must be created before and after the ontology translation; e.g., creating specific metaclasses, transforming sets of components in a simpler one, adding specific pieces of documentation to ontology components transformed, etc. Finally, also in this layer we may decide, in case the target format is an ontology tool, which transformations have to be made to the user interface to comply with the pragmatic properties determined during the analysis activity (we will show examples of these transformations in chapter 4).

Input products and output results

Input: Catalogue of translation decisions to be reused, ontology translation decision scope, and refined requirement catalogue.

Output: Catalogue of translation decisions at the pragmatic level.

Participants

Knowledge and software engineers.

Techniques

Cataloguing and translation decision tables and diagrams.

Practical example

As stated in the functional requisite Req1, the ontology translation system to be developed will be mainly driven by pragmatics; that is, the ontologies must be readable enough both for human users and OWL-aware systems once they have been transformed.

Taking into account this requisite, our first decision has consisted in not transforming some WebODE ontology components that have not a direct correspondence in OWL DL, although they could be represented by means of workarounds. The only exception to this requisite is the transformation of WebODE exhaustive decompositions and partitions of concepts, which will be transformed even when there are not specific OWL DL primitives to represent them.

The second decision is related to the differences in the scope of instance attributes/datatype properties and ad hoc relations/object properties between WebODE and OWL DL. In section 3.2.5 we have already presented some translation possibilities related to this aspect. The following translation decisions are made in the WebODE export service to OWL DL, as summarized in the decision tree of figure 3.10:

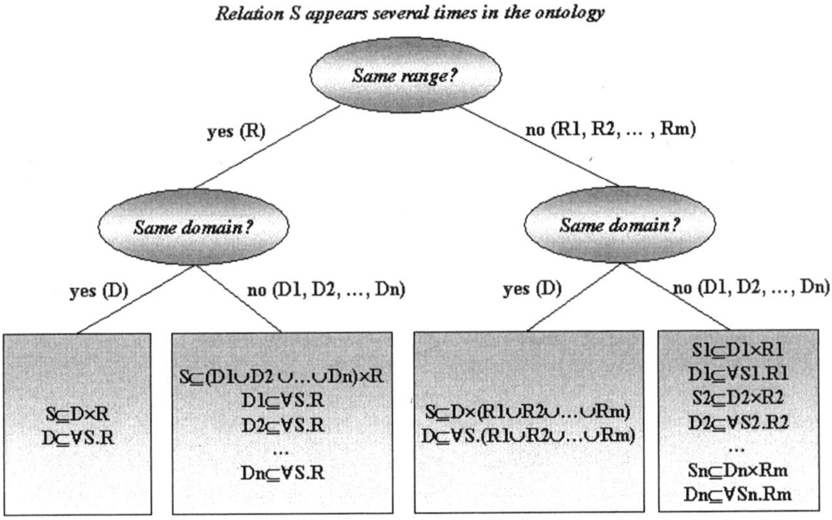

Figure 3.10. Translation decisions taken for transforming the scope of WebODE ad hoc relations

- If several WebODE ad hoc relations or instance attributes have the same name, the same range R, and different domains (D1, D2, ..., Dn), then we consider that they refer to the same OWL object property or datatype property, whose range is R and whose domain is $D1 \cup D2 \cup \ldots \cup Dn$.
- If several WebODE ad hoc relations have the same name, the same domain D, and different ranges (R1, R2, ..., Rn), then we consider that they refer to the same OWL object property, whose domain is D and whose range is $R1 \cup R2 \cup \ldots \cup Rn$. This decision contrasts with what could be interpreted in OWL if these domain and range definitions were expressed independently ($R1 \cap R2 \cap \ldots \cap Rn$).
- If two WebODE ad hoc relations or instance attributes have the same name, but not the same domain nor the same range, then we consider that they refer to different OWL object properties or datatype properties respectively.

The third decision is related to the treatment of the class unions generated as a consequence of the previous transformations. For pragmatic reasons, complex domains and ranges can be post-processed to obtain simpler expressions, so that if for any $Ci \in C$, it holds that $Ci \subseteq C \backslash Ci$, then Ci can be removed from the expression.

Task 3.3. Propose Transformations at the Semantic Level

Similarly to the previous task, in this task we must propose the transformations required to comply with the restrictions related to the semantic preservation properties of the transformation. As with the pragmatic restrictions, the semantic ones were imposed during the analysis activity and described in the refined catalogue of requirements and in the ontology translation decision scope document.

This task will be performed by knowledge engineers, who will describe in detail the transformations needed by means of diagrams and tables. According to the top-down approach described for the design activity, this task will be the second to begin, although it will be performed in parallel. Besides, figure 3.9 suggests that this task will require more effort (both in terms of time and of resources), since this part is the most complex of the ontology translation system design.

To specify the transformations at this layer, we recommend using the same techniques than in the previous task, that is, we recommend using tables and diagrams to specify the relationships between the ontology components in the source and target formats. Based on our experience, we assume that in this layer we will find more translation decisions to be reused from other translation systems. Besides, we will use the results of the tasks 2.1, 2.2 and 2.3 (used to describe the source and target formats, and to determine and to compare their expressiveness) as an input of this task. This input will help to specify these translation decisions.

Input products and output results

Input: Catalogue of translation decisions to be reused, ontology translation decision scope, refined requirement catalogue, KR ontologies of source and target formats, and source and target format comparison.

Output: Catalogue of translation decisions at the semantic level.

Participants

Knowledge and software engineers.

Techniques

Cataloguing and translation decision tables and diagrams.

Practical example

There are many translation decisions that can be made in the semantic layer. As an example, we will show the proposal for transforming a WebODE concept partition into a class equivalence between the parent class and the union of all the subclasses, several subclass of relationships between the subclasses and the parent class, and disjointness axioms between each pair of classes in the partition. This transformation has already been identified in the refined requisite catalogue (and more specifically, in table 3.9).

The design of this transformation is shown in table 3.11 which shows the knowledge found in the source format (WebODE), and its exact correspondence in the target format (OWL DL).

Table 3.11. Semantic transformation of WebODE partitions to OWL DL.

WebODE	**OWL DL**
Partition (C, {C1,C2,...,Cn})	$C \equiv C1 \cup C2 \cup \ldots \cup Cn$ $Ci \subseteq C$ $\quad \forall\, Ci \in \{C1,C2,\ldots,Cn\}$ $Ci \cap Cj \subseteq \bot$ $\quad \forall\, Ci \neq Cj,, Ci,Cj \in \{C1,C2,\ldots,Cn\}$

Task 3.4. Propose Transformations at the Syntax Level

The objective of this task is to propose the transformations to be performed at the syntax layer, so as to overcome the inherently different syntaxes of the source and target formats. Consequently, this task consists in determining which are the syntactic restrictions of the source and target formats, which is the syntax to be used to express each ontology component specified in the previous tasks, and which are other specific correspondences between the source and target formats (e.g., correspondences in the datatypes used, in the information needed for the ontology headers, etc.).

Unlike the previous two tasks, this task can be performed by a software engineer, since it does not have much to do with the knowledge represented and with its intended meaning, but with how this knowledge is represented physically. To perform this task, several techniques can be used: translation decision tables and diagrams (e.g., for specifying the correspondences between datatypes); BNF grammars of the source and target formats (either for all the language expressions or for part of them) to gain more understanding of how each component is represented, of how we should read expressions in the source format and of how we should generate expressions in the target format; and API descriptions of the source and target formats, in case they are available. As we will see later, during the implementation activity, we will force the source and target formats to provide an ontology management API, so that the transformations can be implemented more easily in the ODESyntax language described there. However, this constraint should not be considered yet at this step.

Input products and output results

Input: Catalogue of translation decisions to be reused, ontology translation decision scope, and refined requirement catalogue.

Output: Catalogue of translation decisions at the syntax level.

Participants

Software and knowledge engineers.

Techniques

Cataloguing, translation decision tables and diagrams, and BNF diagrams.

Practical example

The following examples show how to design transformations at the syntax level in the WebODE export service to OWL DL.

Table 3.12 shows the correspondence between the datatypes used for instance attributes in WebODE and the datatypes used in OWL DL.

Table 3.12. WebODE and OWL DL datatype correspondences.

WebODE datatypes	OWL DL datatypes
Boolean	&xsd;boolean
Cardinal	&xsd;nonNegativeInteger
Integer	&xsd;integer
Float	&xsd;float
String	&xsd;string
Date	&xsd;date
Range	&xsd;float
URL	&xsd;anyURI
XML Schema datatype x	x if $x \in$ [built-in XML Schema datatypes] &xsd;string otherwise

As another example of the documentation used in this task, we now show the description of the WebODE API for concept management, and an excerpt of the BNF grammar of OWL DL (in abstract syntax) for class generation.

WebODE API. Concept management

getConcept(ontology,concept):Concept

getChildConcepts(ontology,concept):Concept[]

getParentConcepts(ontology,concept):Concept[]

getGroups(ontology):Group[]

getRootConcepts(ontology):Concept[]

isSubclassOf(ontology,concept1,concept2):boolean

getConceptsInWhichAttributeIsDefined(ontology,attribute):Concept[]

OWL DL Abstract syntax for concept generation

axiom ::= 'Class(' **classID** ['Deprecated'] **modality** { **annotation** } { **description** } ')'

modality ::= 'complete' | 'partial'

description ::= **classID**

| **restriction**

| 'unionOf(' { **description** } ')'

| 'intersectionOf(' { **description** } ')'

| 'complementOf(' **description** ')'

| 'oneOf(' { **individualID** } ')'

Task 3.5. Propose Transformations at the Lexical Level

This is the last task of this group. Its objective is to propose the transformations to be performed at the lexical level to overcome the differences between how the source and target formats express ontology component identifiers, natural language descriptions, and attribute values.

As in the previous task, this task can be performed by software engineers, who may use translation decision tables and diagrams, and BNF grammars of the ontology component identifiers, natural language documentation, and attribute values. In this layer the reuse of translation decisions is very common, since there are not many differences between different formats at this level.

As described in section 3.2.1, the most common problems to solve in this layer refer to the differences about the legal and illegal characters of the source and target formats, and about the scope of ontology components (some ontology components are defined inside the scope of others in one format, while their correspondent ontology components are defined outside their scope).

Input products and output results

Input: Catalogue of translation decisions to be reused, ontology translation decision scope, and refined requirement catalogue.

Output: Catalogue of translation decisions at the lexical level.

Participants

Software and knowledge engineers.

Techniques

Cataloguing, translation decision tables and diagrams, and BNF grammars.

Practical example

The design of transformations at the lexical level in the WebODE export service to OWL DL are reused from the WebODE export service to DAML+OIL. There are specially three types of transformations to be highlighted at this level:

- OWL ontology component identifiers must be valid namespace-qualified names (QNames), which usually consists of two parts: a namespace and a local name, which in its turn must be an NCName [Bray et al., 2000]. Therefore, the ontology translation system must transform WebODE ontology components into QNames by prefixing all the components with the ontology namespace, and by ensuring that the ontology component identifier is transformed to a valid QName. The BNF grammar shown below [Bray et al., 2000] describes how to generate valid QNames:

```
[6]  QName ::= (Prefix ':')? LocalPart
[7]  Prefix ::= NCName
[8]  LocalPart ::= NCName
[4]  NCName ::= (Letter | '_') (NCNameChar)*    /*An XML Name, minus the ":" */
[5]  NCNameChar ::= Letter | Digit | '.' | '-' | '_' | CombiningChar | Extender
[84] Letter  ::=  BaseChar | Ideographic
[85] BaseChar  ::=  [#x0041-#x005A] | [#x0061-#x007A] | [...] | [#xAC00-#xD7A3]
[86] Ideographic  ::=  [#x4E00-#x9FA5] | #x3007 | [#x3021-#x3029]
[87] CombiningChar  ::=  [#x0300-#x0345] | [...] | [#x302A-#x302F] | #x3099 | #x309A
[88] Digit  ::=  [#x0030-#x0039] | [...] | [#x0F20-#x0F29]
```

- The scope of some ontology components is different in the source and in the target formats, as explained in the pragmatic level (task 3.2). The transformations proposed in that section are implemented at the lexical level.
- In WebODE, concepts and instance attributes can share the same identifier, while in OWL DL the sets of identifiers of classes and datatype properties are disjoint. Consequently, if a WebODE concept *Name* and a WebODE instance attribute *Name* have to be transformed into OWL DL, two different identifiers will be generated for them; for example, *Name* and *Name_1* respectively.

Task 3.6. Propose Additional Transformations

Finally, in this task we must propose transformations not taken into account by any of the preceding tasks, either because it was not easy to classify in any of the translation layers or because it is more related to the integration of the ontology translation system generated in other information systems (normally, in other ontology tools).

This task will be performed by software engineers, who must take into account the software and integration restrictions of the resulting ontology translation system. We recommend the use of different techniques to specify these transformations: catalogues of design specifications to be taken into account in the implementation, translation decision tables and diagrams, as in the previous cases, or general design techniques such as class and interaction diagrams (we recommend using design patterns for this [Larman, 2001]), database design specifications, etc.

Input products and output results

Input: Catalogue of translation decisions to be reused, ontology translation decision scope, refined requirement catalogue, and catalogues of translation decisions at the pragmatic, semantic, syntax and lexical levels.

Output: Catalogue of additional transformations.

Participants

Software and knowledge engineers.

Techniques

Cataloguing, translation decision tables and diagrams, database design specifications, design class and interaction diagrams, design patterns, etc.

Practical example

The ontology translation system between WebODE and OWL DL must be integrated as a service in the WebODE platform. To achieve this goal, once the code of the system has been generated, it should be wrapped as a stateless service in the application server underlying the WebODE platform. Figure 3.11 shows the class diagram that corresponds to the classes and interfaces needed to integrate the translation system as a WebODE export service. There are four classes, in charge of the service description and management (*OWLExportServiceManager*), the service configuration (*OWLExportServiceConfiguration*), the service interface (*OWLExportService*), and the service implementation (*OWLExportServiceImp*). The *exportOntology* method of this class will call the necessary methods of the ontology translation service in order to perform the actual translation of ontologies, and will use the *ODEService* interface to access WebODE ontologies.

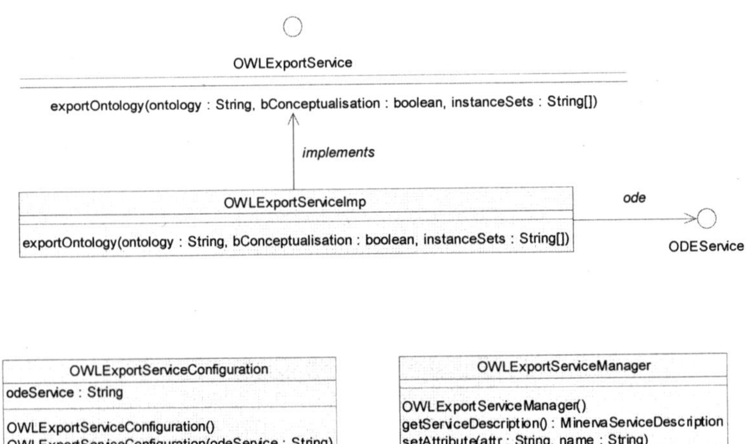

Figure 3.11. Classes and interfaces needed to integrate the ontology translation system as a WebODE export service.

3.4.4 Activity 4. Implementation of the Translation System

The objective of the implementation activity is to create the declarative specifications of the transformations to be performed by the ontology translation system, which will be used to generate its final code. These declarative specifications are based on the results of the design activity (the ontology translation system design) and are implemented in the ODEDialect set of languages: ODELex, ODESyntax, and ODESem, which correspond to the lexical, syntax, and semantic/pragmatic ontology translation layers, respectively.

As in the design activity, the tasks inside this implementation activity are divided into groups, four in this case, as shown in figure 3.12. We describe next the goals and the responsible for each task, which are summarized in table 3.13:

The goal of the unique task of the first group is to select reusable pieces of code from the declarative specifications of other ontology translation systems. These pieces of code are selected on the basis of the results obtained from the first task of the design activity, and can be related to any of the four translation layers. As it occurred in the corresponding task of the design activity, this task is performed by knowledge and software engineers, who focus on different aspects of the existing translation systems. They will catalogue the pieces of code to be reused so that they will find them easily in the following implementation tasks.

The five tasks in the second group should be performed almost in parallel, as shown in the figure. In these tasks the software and knowledge engineers must actually implement the transformations at the four layers: lexical, syntax, semantic, and pragmatics; and the additional transformations described in task 3.6. Unlike in the design activity, we propose to start with the low-level transformations (those at the lexical and syntax layers), and continue with the more abstract (and difficult) ones. The reason for this order is that the implementations of semantic and pragmatic transformations usually need to take into account the specific implementations at the lexical and syntax layers.

The third group contains task 4.7 (declarative specification processing and integration), where the software engineer is in charge of transforming the previous declarative implementations at all levels, plus the additional transformations, into actual running code, which will perform the translations as specified in the previous code. The software engineer must also integrate the resulting ontology translation system into another information system (such as an ontology tool), if required. Given that most of the transformations have been implemented in formal languages, and that the additional transformations have been specified in Java, most of the processes involved in this task can be automated. If problems are detected during this task, the method recommends to solve them going back to the implementation activities.

Finally, the method proposes to execute the test suite defined during the analysis activity, considered as the system test suite for the translation system. This does not prevent us from defining and executing other kinds of tests (from unitary tests to integration tests) at any point during the development. This task consists in inputting the ontologies in the test suite into the resulting ontology translation system and checking whether the output corresponds to the one expected. Note that in most cases this check will consist in comparing whether the output file(s) and the expected file(s) are identical, but there are cases where this kind of comparison will not be possible, since the results can come in any order (for instance, in RDF and OWL ontologies). If any of the test fails, we must go back to the previous implementation activities to detect the problems. Furthermore, we must consider that the method allows moving to previous activities if problems are detected at any point of our development.

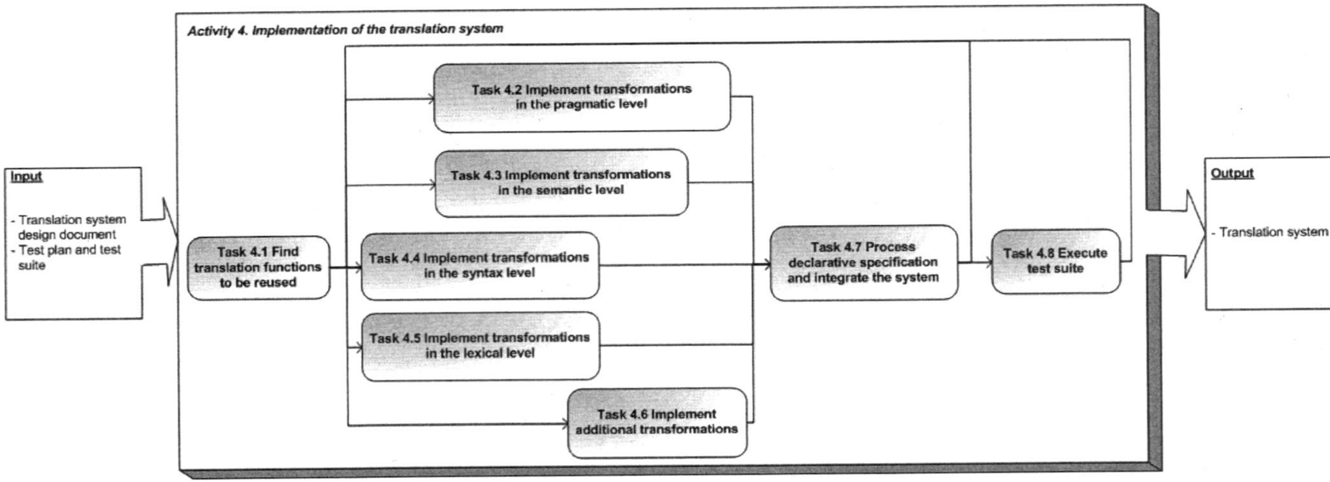

Figure 3.12. Task decomposition of activity 4 (implementation of the translation system).

Task	*Products*	*Techniques*	*Participants*
Task 4.1. Find and reuse similar translation systems	Catalogue of translation functions to be reused	Cataloguing	Software engineer Knowledge engineer
Task 4.2. Propose transformations at the pragmatic level	ODESem implementation	ODESem	Knowledge engineer Software engineer
Task 4.3. Propose transformations at the semantic level	ODESem implementation	ODESem	Knowledge engineer Software engineer
Task 4.4. Propose transformations at the syntactic level	ODESyntax implementation	ODESyntax	Software engineer Knowledge engineer
Task 4.5. Propose transformations at the lexical level	ODELex implementation	ODELex	Software engineer Knowledge engineer
Task 4.6. Propose additional transformations	Additional transformations implementation		Software engineer Knowledge engineer
Task 4.7. Process declarative specification and integrate the system	Java source code Integrated translation system		Software engineer
Task 4.8. Execute test suite	Test results Corrective actions	System tests	Software engineer Knowledge engineer

Table 3.13. Task products, techniques and participants of activity 4 (implementation of the translation system).

Task 4.1. Find Translation Functions to be Reused

In this task we select the pieces of code that will be reused from other ontology translation systems. These pieces of code may include parts of their declarative specifications or user-defined functions. The input for this task is the catalogue of reusable translation decisions obtained as a result of its counterpart task during the design activity (task 3.1).

The pieces of code obtained may belong to any of the four ontology translation layers and will be inserted in the corresponding layer in the next implementation tasks. The selection is performed by software and knowledge engineers, who focus on different aspects of the reuse, as occurred during the design.

Input products and output results

Input: translation system design document (catalogue of translation decisions to be reused).

Output: catalogue of translation functions to be reused.

Participants

Software and knowledge engineer.

Techniques

Cataloguing.

Practical example

In task 3.1 we identified two translation systems from which we could reuse many translation and software design decisions: the WebODE export services to RDF(S) and DAML+OIL. The objective of this task is to select the exact pieces of code that will be reused, so they can be used in the next implementation tasks. We will show some of the reusable pieces of code selected from the DAML+OIL export service:

With regard to translation decisions, one of the aspects to be reused is the transformation of the scope of instance attributes and ad hoc relations (from local to concepts to global to the ontology). As expressed elsewhere, this transformation can be done in at least two different ways: by creating an identifier for each of them, or by trying to find commonalities in their domain and ranges and building complex expressions from them. We will opt for the second way, which was also implemented in the export service to DAML+OIL, and we will reuse the following piece of code from the ODELex specification of that export service.

```
%WebODE.InstanceAttribute IDENTIFIER WebODE.Concept IDENTIFIER WebODE.Type IDENTIFIER
  INIT:       {$1=convertToURI(%1)}
  TABLE:      {([WebODE.InstanceAttribute,%1,%2,%3],[OWL.DatatypeProperty,$1])}
  REPEATED: {[WebODE.InstanceAttribute,%1,_,%3] ==>
                                         {$1=get([WebODE.InstanceAttribute,%1,_,%3])},
             default ==> {$1=addNumber($1)}}
  OVERLAP: {$1=addNumber($1)}

%WebODE.AdHocRelation IDENTIFIER WebODE.Concept IDENTIFIER WebODE.Concept IDENTIFIER
  /* The 2nd and 3rd identifiers are of the domain and range concepts */
  INIT:      {$1=convertToURI(%1)}
  TABLE:     {([WebODE.AdHocRelation,%1,%2,%3],[OWL.ObjectProperty,$1])}
  REPEATED: {[WebODE.AdHocRelation,%1,%2,_] ==>
                                            {$1=get([WebODE.AdHocRelation,%1,%2,_])},
            [WebODE.AdHocRelation,%1,_,%3] ==>
                                            {$1=get([WebODE.AdHocRelation,%1,_,%3])},
            default ==> {$1=addNumber($1)}}
  OVERLAP:   {$1=addNumber($1)}
```

With regard to the implementation code, we selected for reuse the process needed to output the files that contain the translated ontology as a ZIP file. The following function is reused from the WebODE export service to DAML+OIL (we only show its signature):

```
private byte[] _writeOntologyAndInstancesToFile
           (String fileDirectory, boolean bConceptualization,
            String[] instanceSets, String namespace)
```

Task 4.2. Implement Transformations in the Pragmatic Level

The objective of this task is to implement the ontology translation decisions proposed at the pragmatic layer. These decisions were included in the translation system design document. The implementation will be coded with ODESem, a language created specifically for this task (and for the semantic layer, as will be described later). In case a transformation cannot be expressed in this language, a general-purpose programming language can be used.

The task will be performed by knowledge and software engineers: the former will implement the transformations in ODESem, and the latter will implement the additional transformations needed. In addition, the pieces of code selected previously will be reused in this task.

Input products and output results

Input: translation system design document (catalogue of translation decisions at the pragmatic level)

Output: ODESem implementation.

Participants

Knowledge and software engineer.

Techniques

ODESem (cf. section 3.3.3).

Practical example

Some pieces of the declarative code required to express the transformations at the pragmatic level for the WebODE export service to OWL DL have been already shown in section 3.3.3.

Task 4.3. Implement Transformations in the Semantic Level

The objective of this task is to implement the ontology translation decisions proposed at the semantic layer, which were included in the translation system design document. The implementation will be mainly coded with ODESem, as it occurred with the implementation of transformations in the pragmatic layer. Furthermore, as in task 4.2, if a transformation cannot be expressed in this language then a general-purpose programming language can be used.

The task will be performed by knowledge and software engineers: the former will implement the transformations in ODESem, and the latter will implement the additional transformations needed. Besides, the pieces of code selected in task 4.1 will be reused.

Input products and output results

Input: translation system design document (catalogue of translation decisions at the semantic level)

Output: ODESem implementation.

Participants

Knowledge and software engineer.

Techniques

ODESem (cf. section 3.3.3).

Practical example

Some pieces of the declarative code needed to express the transformations at the semantic level for the WebODE export service to OWL DL were already shown in section 3.3.3.

Task 4.4. Implement Transformations in the Syntax Level

The objective of this task is to implement the ontology translation decisions proposed at the syntax layer, which were included in the translation system design document. The implementation will be coded with ODESyntax, a language specifically created to implement this type of transformations. As in the previous implementation tasks, if a transformation cannot be expressed in ODESyntax then a general-purpose programming language can be used.

The task will be mainly performed by software engineers, although knowledge engineers can be helpful. Additionally, the pieces of code selected in task 4.1 will be reused.

Input products and output results

Input: translation system design document (catalogue of translation decisions at the syntax level)

Output: ODESyntax implementation.

Participants

Software and knowledge engineer.

Techniques

ODESyntax (cf. section 3.3.2).

Practical example

Some pieces of the declarative code needed to express the transformations at the syntax level for the WebODE export service to OWL DL were already shown in section 3.3.2.

Task 4.5. Implement Transformations in the Lexical Level

The objective of this task is to implement the ontology translation decisions proposed at the lexical layer, included in the translation system design document. The implementation will be mainly coded with ODELex, a language specifically created to implement this type of transformations. As in the previous implementation tasks, if a transformation cannot be expressed in ODELex then a general-purpose programming language can be used.

The task will be mainly performed by software engineers, although knowledge engineers may also help. Besides, the pieces of code selected in task 4.1 will be reused.

Input products and output results

Input: translation system design document (catalogue of translation decisions at the lexical level)

Output: ODELex implementation.

Participants

Software and knowledge engineer.

Techniques

ODELex (cf. section 3.3.1).

Practical example

Some pieces of the declarative code needed to express the transformations at the lexical level for the WebODE export service to OWL DL have been already shown in section 3.3.1.

Task 4.6. Implement Additional Transformations

The objective of this task is to implement the rest of transformations required for the ontology translation system, and which have not been expressed in any of the four previous tasks. These transformations were designed in task 3.6, by means of general-purpose design techniques, and they are implemented with general-purpose implementation techniques.

This task will be mainly performed by software engineers, although knowledge engineers may also help to implement some of the transformations. Besides, pieces of code selected in task 4.1 can be reused.

Input products and output results

Input: translation system design document (catalogue of additional transformations)

Output: Additional transformations implementation (normally, Java code to be appended to the translation system before its integration).

Participants

Software and knowledge engineer.

Techniques

--

Practical example

As a result of this task, the implementation code needed to integrate the ontology translation system as a WebODE export service is generated. We have reused part of the code from the WebODE export service to DAML+OIL.

Task 4.7. Process Declarative Specification and Integrate the System

In this task, the multi-layered declarative implementation of the ontology translation system together with the additional functions that might have been implemented are processed in order to generate the final code of the ontology translation system and to integrate it.

This task is performed by software engineers, who must follow a set of recommendations for generating this final code. Recommendations are different for each layer, since the problems to be solved and the code to be generated in each layer are different and thus they need different programming techniques. Given that most of the transformations have been implemented in formal languages, and that the additional transformations have been specified in Java, most of the processes involved in this task can be automated.

If a problem appears during this task, due to problems in any preceding implementation task, then we must go back to those tasks to solve it.

Input products and output results

Input: translation decision implementations in ODESem, ODESyntax, ODELex, and additional transformations.

Output: Java source code of the ontology translation system, and integrated software.

Participants

Software engineer.

Techniques

ODEDialect.

Practical example

--

Task 4.8. Execute Test Suite

The objective of this task is to determine the correct functioning of the ontology translation system generated and integrated in the previous task. To check the ontology translation system's validity, we will use the test suite defined during the task 2.6 of the analysis activity. This test suite was created as a set of system tests that the system should pass successfully in order to consider it valid. The test suite contains a set of input ontologies in the source format of the ontology translation system and their corresponding output ontologies in the target format. The set usually covers exhaustively the possibilities where the translation system must make translation decisions.

To pass the test, the output ontologies must correspond with the ontologies expected in each case. As we commented in the introduction to this implementation activity, this check will normally consist in comparing whether the output file(s) and the expected file(s) are identical. However, there will be cases where this kind of comparison is not possible, since the results can be generated in any order.

If any of the test fails, we must go back to the previous implementation activities to detect the source of the problems and propose corrective actions. Furthermore, we must consider that the method allows going back to previous activities if problems are detected at any point of our development.

This task must be performed by software and knowledge engineers, since in case of unsuccessful cases they have to detect the sources of the problems detected and propose the corrective actions.

Input products and output results

Input: integrated ontology translation system, test plan and test suite.

Output: test results and proposed corrective actions.

Participants

Software and knowledge engineer.

Techniques

Test systems.

Practical example

The result of task 2.6 was a test plan containing a test suite with synthetic ontologies. These ontologies had to be used to check the conformance of the WebODE export service to OWL DL to the transformation results expected. An example of one of the errors found when running these tests, and the corrective action taken to solve it, is shown below:

One of the WebODE ontologies included in the test contained the concept *C*, the instance attribute *C* defined in the concept *C* and with datatype *String*, and the instance *C* of concept *C*. This is possible in WebODE since the sets of identifiers for these ontology components are not necessarily disjoint, though they refer to different components. The expected result of the test was a class, a datatype property and an instance, all of them with different identifiers (e.g., C, C_1, and C_1_1 respectively).

The first time the test was run, we discovered that there were only two different identifiers, because the concept and the instance had the same identifier. This is not valid OWL DL, but OWL Full, and hence it was the result of an incorrect transformation. We analyzed the lexical transformation code from the ontology translation system and we discovered that we had not explicitly stated that there could not be overlap between OWL class identifiers and OWL individual identifiers. Hence the proposed corrective action was to express explicitly that "no-overlapping" relationship; the next time that the test was executed it passed successfully.

Chapter 4
Semantic and Pragmatic Preservation in Ontology Translation

This chapter presents four approaches used so far in ontology translation, taking into account the two perspectives related to the semantic and pragmatic ontology translation layers. The chapter describes how these approaches preserve the knowledge represented in an ontology and its intended meaning when this ontology is transformed from one format into another. These descriptions put special emphasis on the lifecycle of knowledge in cyclic ontology translation processes.

4.1 Transformation Approaches and their Implications in Semantic and Pragmatic Preservation

The ontology translation model proposed in this document considers that ontology translation problems can appear, and hence they have to be solved, at four different but interrelated layers: lexical, syntax, semantic, and pragmatic. The problems that appear at these four layers are equally important and all of them must be solved to allow transforming an ontology successfully from the source into the target format. However the decisions made at the semantic and pragmatic layers are those that usually drive the transformations to be performed by the ontology translation system.

The overall objective of an ontology translation system is often to obtain an ontology in the target format with maximal preservation properties in each of the four previous ontology translation layers.

Let τ be a transformation function between the formats L and L' (τ:L→L') that is implemented by an ontology translation system. At each translation level, we can consider the following maximal preservation properties (adapted from [Euzenat, 2001]):

- At the lexical layer, *synset preservation* (a synset is the set of connected components of the synonymy graph S). That is, $\forall t,t' \in L, S(t) = S(t') \Rightarrow S(\tau(t)) = S(\tau(t'))$.
- At the syntactic level, *order preservation*. That is, given two order relations for the formats L and L' ($\leq_L$ and $\leq_{L'}$ respectively), $\forall r,s \in L, r \leq_L s \Rightarrow \tau(r) \leq_{L'} \tau(s)$.
- At the semantic level, *consequence preservation*. That is, $\forall r,\delta \in L, r \models_L \delta \Rightarrow \tau(r) \models_{L'} \tau(\delta)$
- At the pragmatic level, *interpretation preservation*. That is, let Σ be the interpretation rules, P the set of persons or systems that must interpret the expressions defined in the

format L, and $\models^i$ the interpretation relation for person or system i, $\forall r,\delta \in L, \forall i,j \in P$, $(r,\Sigma \models^i \delta \Rightarrow \tau(r),\tau(\Sigma) \models^j \tau(\delta))$.

However, in many cases not all of these maximal preservation properties can be achieved simultaneously in an ontology translation system, since there is usually an important trade-off among the preservation properties that can be obtained at each layer. For instance, it is not always easy to achieve maximum semantic preservation (consequence preservation) and maximum pragmatic preservation (intended meaning or interpretation preservation) at the same time. Let us show an example of a transformation from the ontology language OWL DL to the ontology tool Protégé-2000 in order to illustrate this trade-off:

Let us suppose that we have an OWL DL ontology with the class `Person` and the object property `hasParents`, whose domain is `Person`, whose cardinality is 2, and whose range is the union of the classes `Man` and `Woman`. Besides, the class `Person` has two existential restrictions regarding this property, stating that any instance of this class must be connected at least to one instance of the class `Man`, and to one instance of the class `Woman`. In the DL formalism, this is expressed as follows:

$$\text{Person} \subseteq (\geq 2\ \text{hasParents}) \cap (\leq 2\ \text{hasParents}) \cap (\forall \text{hasParents}.(\text{Man} \cup \text{Woman})) \cap$$
$$(\exists \text{hasParents}.\text{Man}) \cap (\exists \text{hasParents}.\text{Woman})$$

There are at least two alternatives to transform this expression to Protégé-2000:

- Preserving the semantics of the original expression while making the expression difficult to understand in the target format by human users and applications. We create the slot `hasParents` whose domain is the class `Person`, whose range is the class `ManOrWoman`, and whose cardinality is 2. This slot is attached to the class `Person`. The class `ManOrWoman` is declared as an abstract class, with the classes `Man` and `Woman` as its subclasses. Besides, we create an additional PAL constraint stating that if an instance of the class `Person` has two values for the slot `hasParents`, one of them is instance of the class `Man` and the other is instance of the class `Woman`, or vice versa. A diagram of the classes and relations obtained, together with the PAL constraint, is shown in figure 4.1.

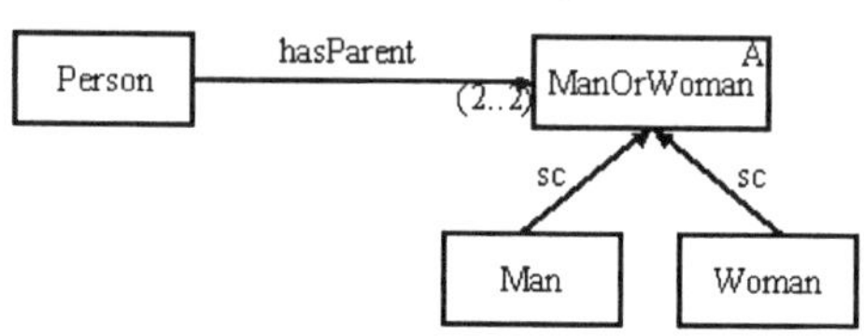


```
(forall ?X (forall ?Y (foralll ?Z
    (=> (and (hasParent ?X ?Y)(hasParent ?X ?Z)(\= ?Y ?Z))
        (or (and (instance-of ?Y Man)(instance-of ?Z Woman))
            (and (instance-of ?Y Woman)(instance-of ?Z Man)))))))
(defrange ?X :FRAME Person)
(defrange ?Y :FRAME ManOrWoman)
(defrange ?Z :FRAME ManOrWoman)
```

Figure 4.1. Semantic preserving transformation of the class `Person` and of the object property `hasParents` from OWL DL to Protégé-2000.

- Not preserving the exact semantics of the original expression, while making the transformed ontology easy to understand. We create two additional slots: `hasFather` (with domain `Person` and range `Man`) and `hasMother` (with domain `Person` and range `Woman`), both of them subslots of the slot `hasParent` and both of them with cardinality 1. These slots are attached to the class `Person`, as shown in figure 4.2.

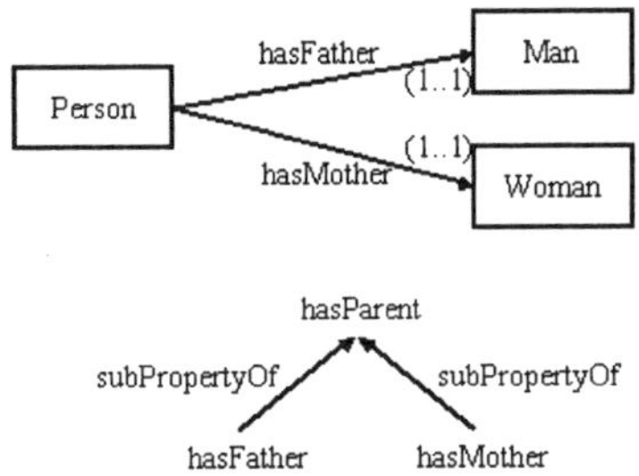

Figure 4.2. Pragmatic preserving transformation of the class `Person` and the object property `hasParents` from OWL DL to Protégé-2000.

One of these alternatives has to be selected for transforming the OWL DL ontology into Protégé-2000. The selection to be made usually depends on the preservation properties needed for the ontology translation system: maximal preservation in the semantic layer or in the pragmatic layer.

In this chapter we explore different approaches used for ontology translation between heterogeneous formats, and comment on their main advantages and disadvantages from the points of view of semantic and pragmatic preservation. Special attention is paid to the preservation of the semantics and of the intended meaning of knowledge in cyclic transformations, that is, transformations where ontologies are finally obtained in the source format after combining several intermediate transformations.

This analysis is included as a separate chapter of this book instead of being included as part of the state of the art, because it presents a deep analysis and comparison of the four translation approaches from the perspectives of semantic and pragmatic preservation, hence contributing to the current state of the art.

The four alternatives explored are:

- Indirect ontology translation between the source and target formats by means of common interchange formats (section 4.2). More specifically, we explore the use of KIF (section 4.2.1), RDF(S) (section 4.2.2), and OWL (section 4.2.3).
- Direct ontology translation between the source and target formats without using additional components or workarounds for representing the knowledge that cannot be directly represented in the target format (section 4.3.1).
- Direct ontology translation between the source and target formats by instantiating the source format KR ontology in the target format (section 4.3.2).
- Direct ontology translation between the source and target formats by using the knowledge components of the target format as much as possible, and by using only additional components or workarounds for representing the knowledge that cannot be directly represented in the target format (section 4.3.3).

4.2 Indirect Ontology Translation by means of Common Interchange Formats

In the beginning of the 1990s, several standard knowledge representation formats were proposed to exchange knowledge between heterogeneous systems. Among them we can cite: CKRL (Common Knowledge Representation Language) [Morik et al., 1991] for exchanging knowledge between machine learning tools; EXPRESS [Spiby, 1992] for exchanging product descriptions; SUMM (Semantic Unification Meta-Model) [Fulton et al., 1992] for enterprise integration; KIF (Knowledge Interchange Format) [Genesereth and Fikes, 1992] for exchanging knowledge between generic knowledge representation systems; PIF (Process Interchange Format) [Lee et al., 1998] for exchanging knowledge about processes; KRSL (Knowledge Representation Specification Language) [Allen and Lehrer, 1992] for exchanging knowledge about planning, etc.

A common feature of most of the aforementioned knowledge exchange languages (aka common interchange languages or interlinguas) is that they were not created nor intended to be used as the internal format of KR systems; they were created for knowledge communication and exchange tasks. Another common feature is that these standardization efforts were aimed at reducing the number of translators needed to achieve interoperability among a heterogeneous group of languages or systems (from $O(n^2)$ to $O(n)$ translators for a number n of systems). This approach corresponds to the pivot architecture described in section 1.5.

Recently, the World Wide Web Consortium (W3C) has proposed three languages as recommendations of the emerging Semantic Web, namely RDF [Lassila and Swick, 1999], RDF Schema [Brickley and Guha, 2004], and OWL [Dean and Schreiber, 2004]. As described in chapter 1, these languages have been created with the purpose of becoming standards for knowledge representation in the Semantic Web. As a consequence, they can be considered as potential common exchange languages, although this is not their main objective.

Given our focus on the ontology field, in this section we will only describe and analyze the use of KIF, RDF(S) (the combination of RDF and RDF Schema), and OWL as common knowledge interchange formats. There are two main advantages in using them for ontology translation processes. First, the number of translation systems needed to transform ontologies between two formats is reduced. Second, if the source and target formats provide export and import services to and from any of these interlinguas, the implementation effort needed to perform the ontology translation is dramatically reduced.

Taking into account the previous consideration, we will describe the main advantages and disadvantages of each format, with examples of how actual translation systems translate to and from these formats. In our analysis of the semantic and pragmatic preservation properties of this approach, we will show that in these interchange formats there is a trade-off between being strict enough to allow exchanging ontologies easily and being extensible enough to ensure knowledge preservation.

4.2.1 KIF as an Interchange Format

As described in chapter 1, the KIF language was developed at the beginning of the 1990s to facilitate knowledge sharing. KIF's main features were its declarative semantics and its provision for expressing arbitrary sentences in first order logic, using four kinds of expressions: terms, sentences, rules, and definitions.

Despite its development as an interchange format, **KIF has not been widely used in ontology exchange between ontology tools and languages**. The tool interoperability tables appearing in [Gómez-Pérez, 2002] confirm that after one decade of KIF existence there are only two ontology tools able to translate ontologies to and from KIF: the Ontolingua Server and OntoSaurus. Besides, WebOnto translates ontologies to Ontolingua, which can be transformed later to KIF by the Ontolingua Server; however, WebOnto does not import Ontolingua nor KIF ontologies. The main conclusion to be extracted from this lack of translation systems is that KIF has not succeeded as a *de facto* standard in the ontology community. Let us see some of the reasons for this lack of success.

1. **KIF allows representing the same knowledge in many different ways, making knowledge exchange difficult**. There are many examples that show this problem, derived from the flexibility of KIF's knowledge model. For instance, the subclass relationship between the classes A and B can be stated with the following two expressions:

```
(Subclass-Of A B)
(=> (A ?x) (B ?x))
```

The first expression uses the relation *Subclass-Of* between the classes A and B. The second expression, which is equivalent, expresses that an instance of the class A is also an instance of the class B[32].

[Pease et al., 2000] show a more complex example related to how to express the type of the KIF variables used inside a KIF expression:

(1) With KIF-style typed quantifiers, before the KIF expression:

(forall ((?x Class1) (?y Class2)) ...)

(2) With *instance-of* relations, inside the KIF expression:

(forall (?x ?y) (and (instance-of ?x Class1) (instance-of ?y Class2)...))

(3) With predicates whose name is the class to which the variable belongs, inside the KIF expression:

(forall (?x ?y) (and (Class1 ?x) (Class2 ?y) ...)).

The flexibility to express the same knowledge in many different ways causes many ontology translation problems, especially during the process of importing ontologies from the interlingua. To solve these, it is usually advisable to accompany knowledge exchange standards by a style guide that imposes how to represent specific pieces of knowledge in the interlingua for exchange purposes. For instance, such a style guide may impose that the type of the variables used in KIF axioms must be defined inside the quantifier specification, as in the first of the options presented above.

2. **Translations to KIF are usually written with regard to a specific format**. The current KIF translation systems use the vocabulary of the source format KR ontology in their translations.

As an example, figure 4.3 shows two definitions in Ontolingua and LOOM, which are equivalent. Both of them define the attribute `engine-count` of the concept `Moving-Object`[33]. The attribute type is integer and its cardinality is one (consequently, in Ontolingua it is represented as a function). The figure also shows the corresponding KIF code generated by the Ontolingua Server and OntoSaurus, which have many differences between them.

Each tool generates KIF expressions according to their own vocabularies. The Ontolingua Server generates KIF expressions with the terms *Function*, *Domain*, *Range*, *Arity*, etc.,

---

[32] *Note that* $\forall x\,(A(x) \rightarrow B(x))$ *in classic first order logic does not have exactly the same meaning as Subclass-Of(A,B) in the paradigm of frames. For example, non-monotonic reasoning is usually considered when reasoning with frames, and disregarded in classic first order logic. To learn more about the relationships between frames and first order logic, consult [Brewka, 1987].*

[33] *The LOOM definition is extracted and adapted from the ontology* `Aircraft`*, which is available in the demo version of the OntoSaurus tool.*

which are relations defined in the *Frame Ontology*, and which have their corresponding KIF axioms in that ontology. OntoSaurus generates KIF expressions using "pure" first-order logic expressions, except for the *LOOM:SINGLE-VALUED* expression, which represents the restriction of the relation cardinality to one.

LOOM

```
(defrelation ENGINE-COUNT
 :DOMAIN MOVING-OBJECT
 :RANGE INTEGER
 :CHARACTERISTICS :SINGLE-VALUED)
```

LOOM → KIF

```
(DEFRELATION ENGINE-COUNT (?A ?B)
        (LOOM:SINGLE-VALUED ENGINE-COUNT))
(FORALL (?B) (=> (ENGINE-COUNT ?A ?B) (INTEGER ?B)))
(FORALL (?A) (=> (ENGINE-COUNT ?A ?B) (MOVING-OBJECT ?A)))
```

Ontolingua

```
(Define-Function Engine-Count (?A) :-> ?B
:Def (and (Moving-Object ?A)
          (Integer ?B)))
```

Ontolingua → KIF

```
(deffunction Engine-Count
  (Function Engine-Count)
  (Range Engine-Count Integer)
  (Domain Engine-Count Moving-Object)
  (Arity Engine-Count 2)
  (Function-Arity Engine-Count 1)
  (Binary-Relation Engine-Count))
```

Figure 4.3. Different KIF representations of the same single-valued attribute.

The previous example illustrates a problem that is not only found in translations from the Ontolingua Server and OntoSaurus; this problem is also rather common in KIF translations from other source formats. For instance, Raschid and Vidal [Raschid and Vidal, 1996] describe how they transform F-Logic ontologies into KIF in order to create a KIF mediator to interoperate with multiple databases. The generated KIF expressions use the F-Logic vocabulary: *is-a* predicates to express the *Subclass-Of* relationship, *fun-value* predicates to express the attribute values, etc. The KIF axioms corresponding to these F-Logic-style predicates, which are necessary to deal with the KIF expressions obtained, are also translated into a Meta-Knowledge Base.

In an ideal scenario, KIF theories should be translatable from and to multiple languages. However, in practice, there is a trade-off between the neutrality of KIF translations and their operational use in different operational languages, as shown as a result of the Neutral Representation project [Barley et al, 1997]. If KIF theories are written without regard to a specific source or target language, then the theories become untranslatable and hence of no operational use; on the other hand, if KIF theories are written for a specific source or target language (using only KIF constructs that are easily translatable to and from it) then the translation loses all the benefits of neutrality and the theory's contents will not be correctly delivered to systems based on other languages.

3. **Interoperability with KIF has been only proved with the same origin and target languages**. Translation to and from KIF has been demonstrated for individual languages (LOOM and Ontolingua). For instance, if we translate from Ontolingua to KIF, and then back to Ontolingua, the KIF translation system is able to recognize easily the Ontolingua-based vocabulary previously generated. However, these experiments are of little use to prove the usefulness of KIF for interoperability [Ginsberg, 1991].

As an example, figure 4.4 shows how the Ontolingua Server imports the KIF codes of the attribute `engine-count` from figure 4.3.

```
(DEFRELATION ENGINE-COUNT (?A ?B)
      (LOOM:SINGLE-VALUED ENGINE-COUNT))
(FORALL (?B) (=> (ENGINE-COUNT ?A ?B) (INTEGER ?B)))
(FORALL (?A) (=> (ENGINE-COUNT ?A ?B) (MOVING-OBJECT ?A)))
```

KIF → Ontolingua

```
(Define-Relation Engine-Count (?A ?B)
:Axiom-Constraints
  (and (forall (?B) (=> (Engine-Count ?A ?B) (Integer ?B)))
       (forall (?A) (=> (Engine-Count ?A ?B) (Moving-Object ?A)))))
```

a) Ontolingua definition obtained after importing the KIF code generated from LOOM

```
(deffunction Engine-Count
  (Function Engine-Count)
  (Range Engine-Count Integer)
  (Domain Engine-Count Moving-Object)
  (Arity Engine-Count 2)
  (Function-Arity Engine-Count 1)
  (Binary-Relation Engine-Count))
```

KIF → Ontolingua

```
(Define-Function Engine-Count (?X) :-> ?Result
:Axiom-Def
  (And (Function Engine-Count)
       (Range Engine-Count Integer)
       (Domain Engine-Count Moving-Object)
       (Arity Engine-Count 2)
       (Function-Arity Engine-Count 1)
       (Binary-Relation Engine-Count)))
```

b) Ontolingua definition obtained after importing the KIF code generated from Ontolingua

Figure 4.4. Results of importing to the Ontolingua Server the KIF code generated from LOOM and Ontolingua.

The Ontolingua definition obtained from the LOOM-generated KIF (figure 4.4.a) loses the cardinality knowledge. Besides, the domain and range of `engine-count` are expressed by means of a first order logic axiom; that is, the definition does not use the Ontolingua relations *Domain* and *Range*, as in figure 4.3. Although both definitions express the same knowledge, the one in figure 4.4.a is less readable than the one in figure 4.3.

This problem even appears in the translation of the Ontolingua-generated KIF code into Ontolingua (figure 4.4.b). The relations *Domain* and *Range* are used inside an *:axiom-def* expression (they do not use variables in the expressions, but the function and class names), which is equivalent to the *:def* expression (which uses variables). Other primitives express redundant knowledge, such as *Function*, *Arity*, *Function-Arity*, and *Binary-Relation*.

The reason for these bad results is due to the variety of styles used to generate KIF expressions. This variety makes it difficult for automatic translation systems to recognize the KIF constructs generated by other systems. How can an automatic translation system recognize, for instance, the *Subclass-Of* predicate? What if *is-a* is used instead? Is the translator into the interlingua expected to provide a declarative description of the predicates used (e.g., that *Subclass-Of* is transitive, included in a Meta-Knowledge Base such as in the F-Logic example) and the translator out is supposed to recognize such description?

In summary, all the problems that appear when using KIF as an interchange language are mainly related to the pragmatic layer: KIF was designed to allow representing the knowledge that could be implemented in a wide variety of knowledge representation languages. Due to its flexibility, the same knowledge can be expressed in many different and equivalent ways, what makes it difficult for other systems to understand KIF correctly. Because of this problem in the pragmatic layer, some other problems appear in the semantic layer, that is, some knowledge can be lost in the translation process, especially in the case where the source and target formats are not the same.

4.2.2 RDF(S) as an Interchange Format

In contrast to KIF, [Gómez-Pérez, 2002] shows that **RDF(S) has been widely adopted by ontology tools as an import/export format**. That is, the combination of RDF and RDF Schema has become a *de facto* standard for exchanging ontologies. Furthermore, not only ontology tools have adopted this language combination for ontology exchange, but also other general software tools have adopted RDF(S) as their content exchange format (Internet browsers like Mozilla, search engines and content providers like Amazon, AltaVista, etc.).

However, the availability of RDF(S) export/import services in most of the ontology tools does not mean that these tools can interoperate. In other words, they do not ensure that ontologies can be actually exchanged without modifying manually their source code or without losing knowledge in the translation process. This conclusion was recently reached by the OntoWeb Special Interest Group on Enterprise-Standard Ontology Environments[34], as a result of the interoperability experiment carried out for the ISWC2003 Workshop on Evaluation of Ontology Tools (EON2003)[35] [Sure et al., 2003], and is also presented in [Polikoff and Allemang, 2003].

The experiment consisted in analyzing how ontologies could be exchanged between different tools and/or languages using RDF(S) and/or OWL as interchange formats. The experiment results can be found in [Isaac et al., 2003; Corcho et al., 2003a; Fillies, 2003]. They deal with the following ontology tools: Differential Ontology Editor[36], KAON [Maedche et al., 2003], OilEd [Bechhofer et al., 2001], OntoEdit [Sure et al., 2002], Protégé-2000 [Noy et al., 2000], SemTalk [Fillies et al., 2002], and WebODE [Arpírez et al., 2003]. Let us summarize some of the conclusions that can be extracted from this experiment and from our analysis of the main features of RDF(S):

1. **RDF(S) allows representing the same knowledge in different ways, making knowledge exchange difficult**. RDF(S) documents can be serialized with three different syntaxes: RDF/XML [Beckett, 2004], Notation-3[37] (N3), and its subset N-Triples[38]. The first syntax is intended for machine-consumption and is normative; however, there are several ways to express the same knowledge with this syntax. The second and third are mainly intended for human-consumption. The figure 4.5 shows the definition of the class `A`, which is a subclass of the class `B`, with two different syntaxes for RDF/XML, with Notation-3 and N-Triples.

Abbreviated RDF/XML	<rdfs:Class rdf:ID="A"> <rdfs:subClassOf rdf:resource="#B"/> </rdfs:Class>
RDF/XML	<rdf:Description rdf:about="#A"> <rdf:type rdf:resource="http://www.w3.org/2000/01/rdf-schema#Class"/> <rdfs:subClassOf rdf:resource="#B"/> </rdf:Description>
Notation-3	:A rdf:type rdfs:Class . :A rdfs:subClassOf :B .
N-Triples	<http://examples.org/sampleOntology#A> <http://www.w3.org/1999/02/22-rdf-syntax-ns#type> <http://www.w3.org/2000/01/rdf-schema#Class> <http://examples.org/sampleOntology#A> <http://www.w3.org/2000/01/rdf-schema#subClassOf> <http://examples.org/sampleOntology#B>

Figure 4.5. Different syntaxes used to represent the same knowledge in RDF(S).

---

[34] *http://delicias.dia.fi.upm.es/ontoweb/sig-tools/index.html*

[35] *http://km.aifb.uni-karlsruhe.de/ws/eon2003/*

[36] *http://opales.ina.fr/public/*

[37] *http://www.w3.org/DesignIssues/Notation3.html*

[38] *http://www.w3.org/2001/sw/RDFCore/ntriples/*

Most of the existing RDF(S)-aware APIs and developer tools[39] can manage the previous notations. They can create the object model that corresponds to a RDF(S) ontology, independently of its syntax, and can serialize an object model in at least one of these notations. However, some ontology tools still use RDF(S) source code directly instead of intermediate object models, which cause problems, as shown in [Isaac et al., 2003].

2. **The standard knowledge model of RDF(S) is not expressive enough to represent most of the knowledge that can be represented with existing ontology languages and tools**. As described in chapter 1, the standard RDF(S) knowledge model, also known as "plain RDF(S)", is based on the combination of two knowledge representation paradigms: semantic networks and frames. Plain RDF(S) allows defining classes –organized in class taxonomies– and properties –organized in property hierarchies– with their domain and range. However, plain RDF(S) cannot express types of knowledge that can be represented in many ontology tools and languages, such as cardinality constraints of properties, disjoint and exhaustive knowledge in class taxonomies, first order logic axioms, etc.

For instance, the attribute `engine-count` we dealt with in the previous section is implemented in plain RDF(S), without expressing its cardinality restriction, as follows:

```
<rdf:Property rdf:ID='engine-count'>
  <rdfs:domain rdf:resource='#Vehicle'/>
  <rdfs:range rdf:resource='http://www.w3.org/2001/XMLSchema#integer'/>
</rdf:Property>
```

As a consequence of its limited expressiveness, plain RDF(S) allows exchanging only very lightweight ontologies without losing knowledge in their transformation process. In the case of heavyweight ontologies, much knowledge is lost.

3. **Translations to RDF(S) are usually written taking into account a specific language or tool**. As stated above, if we translate a heavyweight ontology from a more expressive language or tool into plain RDF(S) we will lose knowledge in the resulting RDF(S) ontology. To overcome this problem, two solutions have been proposed up to now. These solutions aim at preserving knowledge in the transformation process through RDF(S):

a) *Represent the knowledge that could be lost inside rdfs:comment tags, using a specific structure for this information.* For instance, plain RDF(S) cannot express class attributes. To preserve this knowledge when translating to RDF(S), [Isaac et al., 2003] propose to represent inside a comment the values of the class attributes of a class: similarity with parent (SWP), similarity with siblings (SWS), difference with siblings (DWS) and difference with parent (DWP). For example, the following comment describes the concept `SpatialEntity` in the travel ontology used in the EON2003 experiment [Isaac et al., 2003]:

```
<rdfs:comment>
  SWP=The entity has a spatio-temporal location
  SWS=The entity is considered mostly in regard of its spatial or
      temporal location
  DWS=The entity is considered mostly in regard of its spatial
      location
  DWP=The entity is considered mostly in regard of its spatial or
      temporal location : The entity is considered mostly in regard of
      its spatial location
</rdfs:comment>
```

[39] *A list of RDF-aware tools can be found at http://www.ilrt.bris.ac.uk/discovery/rdf/resources/*

b) *Extend RDF(S) ontology component descriptions with properties not defined in RDF Schema.* RDF is based on the semantic networks KR paradigm and allows using any label for the graph arcs; these labels do not necessarily belong to the RDF or the RDF Schema vocabularies. Hence we can define the knowledge that could be lost in the translation with specific properties attached to the RDF(S) class and property definitions.

For example, Protégé-2000 implements this solution in its RDF(S) backend. Protégé-2000 users can decide whether to export their ontologies to plain RDF(S) or to a Protégé-specific RDF(S) extension. With the first export format, they lose the knowledge that cannot be represented directly in plain RDF(S): property cardinalities, PAL constraints, etc. With the second, part of the ontology is implemented in plain RDF(S) and the other part is preserved with that extension, as described in [Noy et al., 2001].

For instance, the attribute `engine-count` is exported to Protégé-specific RDF(S) as follows (*a:maxCardinality* corresponds to URI *http://protege.stanford.edu/system#maxCardinality*)[40]:

```
<rdf:Property rdf:about="#engine-count"
              a:maxCardinality="1"
              rdfs:label="engine-count">
   <rdfs:domain rdf:resource="#Vehicle"/>
   <rdfs:range rdf:resource="&rdfs;Literal"/>
</rdf:Property>
```

This case is similar to the KIF case: interoperability with RDF(S) can be easily achieved with the same source and target formats, but it becomes difficult with different source and target formats. For example, KAON provides two different RDF(S) import services: one for plain RDF(S) and another for Protégé RDF(S). In summary, we move back from the situation with O(n) translators to the situation where we needed $O(n^2)$ translators, and thus we lose the main advantages of using a common interlingua.

4. **Current translation systems do still have many errors when exporting and/or importing RDF(S)**. RDF and RDFS have been created rather recently and have evolved during their existence. Besides, related technologies in which RDF and RDFS are based, such as XML namespaces, XML Schema datatypes, etc., have also evolved. As a consequence, some of the existing RDF(S) import and export services are not yet stable enough.

For example, Protégé-2000 uses old namespaces to refer to the RDF and RDFS namespaces [Corcho et al., 2003a; page 108], and transforms attribute datatypes incorrectly.

We can give some more examples regarding the translation of concept and property identifiers [Isaac et al., 2003, Corcho et al., 2003a]. For instance, some translation systems use an incorrect XML encoding for the RDF(S) files when any of the identifiers inside the ontology uses letters with accents; some of them use digits at the beginning of identifiers, which produce incorrect XML URI identifiers, or non allowed symbols like &, :, etc.

In summary, RDF(S) shares most of the problems we identified for KIF: from a pragmatic point of view, there are many possible ways to represent the same knowledge with extensions to the language, and therefore not all the ontology translation systems developed for RDF(S) are able to manage correctly the knowledge generated in this language by other

[40] *The RDF(S) backend for Protégé-2000 does not take into account some of the last modifications of RDF(S), such as the use of XML Schema datatypes, so the type integer is transformed into* &rdfs;Literal.

tools. From a semantic preservation point of view, the expressiveness of RDF(S) is very limited. However, its knowledge model is extensible, and therefore any knowledge can be represented in it, with the problems already identified. Finally, RDF(S) also poses problems in the syntactic level, since it can use different syntaxes to represent the same information, as shown above.

4.2.3 OWL as an Interchange Format

Although OWL was not proposed as a W3C Recommendation until very recently (February 2004), **there are already some early-adopter tools able to manage OWL ontologies**. In contrast to RDF(S), OWL-aware tools are primarily ontology tools (not general tools). The reason for this is that OWL is more complex than RDF(S), whose expressiveness is enough for most of the knowledge exchange needs of the other types of tools.

As occurred with RDF(S), some OWL-aware tools do still present some minor problems when managing this "young" language; problems especially related to namespaces, concept and property identifiers, etc. [Isaac et al., 2003].

As we have done with KIF and RDF(S), we will summarize the main aspects concerned with the use of OWL as an exchange language:

1. **OWL allows representing the same knowledge in different ways, making knowledge exchange difficult**. OWL is built on top of RDF(S), which permits using different syntaxes to express knowledge. Therefore, OWL suffers from the same interoperability problem that we described for RDF(S); and this problem can be solved with OWL-aware APIs and developer tools that abstract the syntax of OWL ontologies.

2. **OWL Lite and OWL DL are not expressive enough to represent some of the knowledge that can be expressed in other ontology languages and tools**. OWL Lite has limited expressiveness: it adds some primitives to RDF(S): cardinality restrictions (restricted to the numbers 0 and 1), object and datatype properties, different types of range restrictions, etc. OWL DL adds some more primitives to OWL Lite: disjointness between classes, union of classes, complement of classes, etc.

However, the knowledge that we can represent with these two sublanguages is restricted in order to ensure the existence of decidable reasoning engines for them. Therefore they are not expressive enough to represent all types of first order logic axioms, which are part of the knowledge models of tools like OntoEdit, Protégé-2000, etc., and of languages like Ontolingua, OCML, F-Logic, etc.

The OWL layered approach allows using OWL Lite and/or OWL DL to express most of the knowledge of the ontology. It ensures an easy ontology exchange between languages and/or tools, provided that the minor problems commented at the beginning of this section are solved. For instance, the attribute `engine-count` would be represented in OWL (both Lite and DL) as follows:

```
<owl:DatatypeProperty rdf:ID='engine-count'>
  <rdf:type rdf:resource='&owl;FunctionalProperty'/>
  <rdfs:domain rdf:resource='#Vehicle'/>
  <rdfs:range rdf:resource='&xsd;integer'/>
</owl:DatatypeProperty>
```

3. **Part of the OWL translations must be written according to a specific format**. To overcome the previous knowledge losses and ensure knowledge preservation in transformations, the OWL Full sublanguage can be used. OWL Full uses the full potential

of RDF(S), what is not permitted in OWL Lite nor OWL DL; that is, OWL Full allows using metaclasses.

Another possible extension is the use of OWL annotation properties to represent this additional knowledge. Annotation properties are not used by OWL inference engines and so they do not affect the reasoning properties of OWL ontologies.

However, as occurred with KIF and RDF(S), the extensions used to represent this additional knowledge depend strongly on the source format, and are not easy to "understand" by the import services of other tools or by ontology translation systems to other languages.

To sum up, OWL is more expressive than RDF(S). Consequently, it allows representing much more knowledge in a standardized way than RDF(S) allowed, and hence the number of problems related to the semantic level is reduced. However, OWL is still less expressive than many other tools, and its extensibility facilities have to be used to avoid losing knowledge in transformations. Nevertheless, these translation solutions are created ad-hoc for specific source or target formats, so using OWL without losing knowledge is difficult. As far as the syntax layer is concerned, OWL has the same problems than RDF(S), although this problem is usually ameliorated by the presence of APIs that abstract the syntax variants of the language.

4.3 Direct Ontology Translation

As shown in the previous section, one of the main advantages of using common interchange formats for translating ontologies between two formats is that they do not usually require additional implementation efforts. This is due to the fact that in many cases there are already ontology translation systems available from the source to the interchange format and vice versa. However, we have shown in the previous section that translations through interchange formats do not usually maintain the semantics nor the pragmatics of the original knowledge.

For this reason, it may be better to implement an ad hoc translation system between the source and the target formats in some cases, following the peer-to-peer translation architecture described in section 1.5. Even though the implementation effort is higher than with the previous pivot approach, the main advantage of building ad-hoc translation systems is that they can take into account the exact translation needs required, which are driven by semantic and pragmatic preservation properties. Consequently, the results obtained with direct transformation approaches are usually better than those obtained with indirect ones.

The following sections describe three types of direct (peer-to-peer) transformation approaches:

- Section 4.3.1 describes direct transformations that use only the components defined in the standard knowledge model of the target format. They consist in transforming only the knowledge that can be expressed with the ontology components available in the standard knowledge model of the target format. With this approach, the translation system does not use any knowledge model extensibility facility that the target format may provide, such as metaclasses, annotation properties, etc. These transformations are mainly driven by pragmatic preservation, but not by semantic preservation.
- Section 4.3.2 describes direct transformations that consist in instantiating the source format KR ontology in the target format. Transformations are performed in two steps:

first, the KR ontology of the source format is created in the target format, as if it were a domain ontology of the target format. Then, ontologies in the source format are translated by creating instances of the KR ontology in the target format. These transformations are mainly driven by semantic preservation, but not by pragmatic preservation.

- Section 4.3.3 describes a hybrid approach. It consists in transforming the ontology components of the source ontology that have a direct correspondence with other ontology components in the target format. The rest of knowledge is transformed into the target format by using its extensibility facilities, such as metaclasses, annotation properties, etc. These transformations are driven by both semantic and pragmatic preservation

For each of these direct transformation approaches we have implemented an ontology translation system between the ontology tools WebODE and Protégé-2000, and vice versa. Their main features will be described in each section.

4.3.1 Direct Translation without Additional Components

This direct transformation approach is the most widely used by the existing ontology translation systems. This approach consists in transforming only the ontology components of the source format that have a direct correspondence with other ontology components of the target format, without using any additional components or workarounds for the source ontology components that cannot be directly transformed. As it will be presented below, this direct approach preserves the pragmatics of the ontology transformed. However, the ontology semantics sometimes is not preserved, depending on the differences in expressiveness of the source and target formats.

To implement such an ad hoc direct translation system, we must first analyze in depth which target ontology components correspond to the source ontology components. Once the mappings between components have been proposed, the transformation process consists in translating each source component into the corresponding one(s) in the target format.

Let us analyze this approach with respect to the preservation of semantics and pragmatics in the transformation:

- With regard to the first aspect (semantic preservation), we can conclude that some knowledge is usually lost in the translation process, unless the source and target formats are very similar. The lost knowledge corresponds to those ontology components that cannot be transformed directly into the target format.
- With regard to the second aspect (pragmatic preservation), the main conclusion reached is that the knowledge transformed is usually legible in the target format, because the components used to represent the target ontology are those belonging to the standard knowledge model of the target format. Obviously, the knowledge that has not been transformed cannot be analyzed from a pragmatic point of view, since it is not present in the target format.

In cyclic transformation processes, the implications of this translation approach are clear: the knowledge finally obtained is the one that can be represented in both the source and the target formats. As a consequence of the first transformation, some knowledge will be lost, as described above. The lost knowledge corresponds to the ontology components of the source format that have not direct correspondences with other ontology components in the target format. In the back-transformation into the original format, there will be no knowledge losses, since the ontology components that are represented in the target format are only those that had a direct correspondence in both formats.

4.3.1.1 Practical Example: from WebODE to Protégé-2000, and vice versa

We have created an ontology translation system that transforms WebODE ontologies into Protégé-2000 ontologies according to the standard knowledge model of Protégé-2000. This means that, in a coarse-grained view, WebODE concepts are transformed into Protégé-2000 classes; WebODE exhaustive decompositions and partitions are transformed into Protégé-2000 class taxonomies and abstract classes; WebODE instance attributes and ad hoc relations are transformed into Protégé-2000 template slots; WebODE class attributes are transformed into Protégé-2000 own slots by means of template slots and metaclasses; and WebODE formal axioms are transformed into Protégé-2000 PAL constraints. The transformations for the translation system from Protégé-2000 into WebODE are inverse to these transformations.

As a result of the transformation of a WebODE ontology into Protégé-2000, the ontology obtained contains all the previous components, but loses completely the knowledge of synonyms and acronyms, bibliographic references, and disjoint knowledge in class taxonomies. In other words, there is not full semantic preservation. Besides, some small pieces of knowledge are also lost, such as those related to attribute datatypes (WebODE URL datatypes and XML Schema datatypes are transformed to the Protégé-2000 *Symbol* datatype), to algebraic properties of relations (such as symmetry, transitiveness, etc.), to the existence of multiple natural language documentations for attributes with the same name, etc. In the back-transformation to WebODE, all the knowledge exported successfully to Protégé-2000 can be transformed back, and the knowledge that was lost is not recovered.

With regard to pragmatics, end users and applications can easily "understand" the ontology obtained, since it uses the standard knowledge model of Protégé-2000: it contains Protégé-2000 classes, slots, PAL constraints, etc. The same applies to the ontology obtained in WebODE as a result of a cyclic transformation.

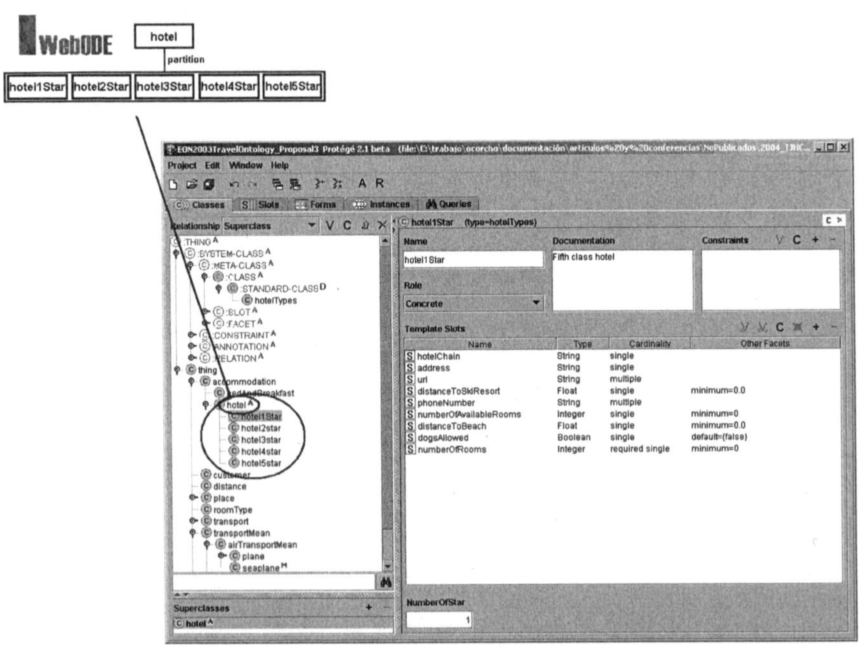

Figure 4.6. Result of a direct translation from WebODE to Protégé-2000 without additional components or workarounds.

Figure 4.6 shows a snapshot of the result of transforming the WebODE travel ontology developed for the EON2002 workshop[41] into Protégé-2000 following this proposal. The figure shows that the concepts `hotel1Star`, `hotel2Star`, `hotel3Star`, `hotel4Star` and `hotel5Star`, which form a partition of the class `hotel` in WebODE, are transformed into Protégé classes that are subclasses of the class `hotel`. In addition, the class `hotel` is defined as an abstract class in Protégé-2000, that is, it cannot have direct instances. The figure also shows that the metaclass `hotelTypes` has been created. This metaclass has the template slot `numberOfStars` attached, which is converted to an own slot in the classes `hotel1Star`, `hotel2Star`, etc., with its corresponding values for each of them (1, 2, etc., respectively)

The previous example is one of the possible approaches for transforming directly a WebODE ontology into Protégé-2000, and vice versa, using their standard knowledge models. Obviously, there are more possibilities that could make use of the standard knowledge models of both ontology tools while making transformations easily understandable for WebODE and Protégé-2000 users.

For instance, since the knowledge models of both tools are based on a combination of frames and first order logic, much knowledge can be expressed by means of first order logic axioms. For example, the previous system would allow creating a class that is a direct or indirect subclass of the classes `hotel1Star` and `hotel2Star` at the same time, what is not correct because those classes are disjoint in the source ontology. To avoid this, a WebODE partition can be transformed not only by creating all the *subclass of* relationships between the classes in the partition and the superclass, and declaring the superclass as abstract, but also by adding PAL constraints stating that all the classes in the partition are disjoint to each other. The following constraint would be added to the class `hotel1Star` (and similarly to the other classes in the partition):

```
(forall ?X
   (=> (subclass-of ?X hotel1Star)
       (and (not (subclass-of ?X hotel2Star))
            (not (subclass-of ?X hotel3Star))
            (not (subclass-of ?X hotel4Star))
            (not (subclass-of ?X hotel5Star))))))
```

This transformation does still use the Protégé-2000 standard knowledge model, although it creates a workaround to represent the disjointness between classes, what is something not directly available in Protégé-2000. However, we may consider that this axiom is still legible by Protégé-2000 users, and hence this type of transformation would fall inside the category of translation approaches described in this section.

4.3.2 Direct Translation by Instantiating the Source Format KR ontology in the Target Format

This approach consists in creating first the KR ontology of the source format in the target one, with the standard knowledge modeling components of the target format, that is, with its concepts or classes, its relations, slots, roles or properties, its formal axioms, etc. Basically, this consists in developing the KR ontology of the source format as if it was a domain ontology of the target format. Once that this KR ontology has been created, the translation process consists in creating instances of that KR ontology according to the contents of the ontology to be transformed. For instance, a concept in the source format is transformed into an instance of the class *Concept* in the target format; an instance in the source format is transformed into an instance of the class *Instance* in the target format, and

[41] *http://km.aifb.uni-karlsruhe.de/eon2002*

is connected to one or several instances of the class *Concept* by means of the relation *isInstanceOf*; etc.

To sum up, the only translation decisions considered in this transformation are related to the lexical and syntax levels of the ontology translation model described in chapter 4. No translation decisions have to be taken in the semantic or the pragmatic layers. Therefore, the transformation process is extremely simple.

The main advantage of this translation approach is that it allows preserving the semantics of the original ontology: all the knowledge inside all the original ontology components is transformed completely into the target format. This approach ensures knowledge preservation in cyclic transformations. That is, if the ontology obtained is back-transformed to the source format, we will finally be able to obtain exactly the same ontology we had originally.

With regard to pragmatics this approach obtains bad results. The KR ontology is created by means of the standard knowledge modeling components of the target format (classes or concepts; relations, roles, slots or properties; formal axioms, etc.), and all the knowledge of the original ontology is transformed into instances of the components represented in that KR ontology. The result is that the ontology transformed into the target format is not legible by human users nor by systems.

However, in cyclic transformations an interesting preservation property arises: the original ontology can be recovered completely when it is back-transformed from the target format. Therefore, we can say that even though the pragmatics of the ontology is not preserved in the transformation into the target format, it is preserved in cyclic transformations.

In conclusion, this approach does not make a real translation of knowledge from one format into another; it basically performs a transformation in the lexical and syntactic layers, avoiding the difficult task of semantic and pragmatic translation. Another drawback of this approach is that the number of ontology translation systems to be developed is double. For example, to perform cyclic transformations between two formats, four translation systems are needed: for cyclic transformations starting in L1, we need a translator from L1 to L2, and another from L2 to L1; for cyclic transformations starting in L2, we need a translator from L2 to L1, and another from L1 to L2.

4.3.2.1 Practical Example: from WebODE to Protégé-2000, and vice versa

To illustrate the ontology translation approach presented in this section, we have implemented another ontology translation system from WebODE into Protégé-2000, and vice versa, starting in WebODE. We have created the WebODE KR ontology by means of Protégé-2000 classes and slots.

This KR ontology contains 14 classes, which represent the ontology components of the WebODE knowledge model: *:WebODEComponent*, *:Concept*, *:Attribute*, *:InstanceAttribute*, *:ClassAttribute*, *:AdHocRelation*, *:Axiom*, *:Instance, :Group*, *:Constant*, *:Property*, *:Synonym*, *:Acronym*, and *:Reference*. The KR ontology also contains 36 slots that represent the relationships between the previous components: *:name*, *:documentation*, *:hasAttribute*, *:hasDomain*, *:hasRange*, *:datatype*, *:maxCardinality*, *:minCardinality*, *:minValue*, *:maxValue*, *:measurementUnit*, *:precision*, *:hasValues*, *:isSubclassOf*, *:isDisjointDecompositionOf*, *:isExhaustiveDecompositionOf*, *:isPartitionOf*, *:hasFormalExpression*, *:isInstanceOf*, etc. Finally, the ontology contains 32 PAL constraints that model restrictions of the WebODE knowledge model.

Figure 4.7 shows a screenshot of the WebODE KR ontology modeled in Protégé-2000. The figure shows the details of the *:InstanceAttribute* class, the slots inherited from its superclasses *:WebODEComponent* and *:Attribute* (*:name*, *:documentation*, *:datatype*, *:minCardinality*, *:maxCardinality*, *:minValue*, *:maxValue*, *:measurementUnit*, and *:precision*), and the slot attached to it: *:hasValues*.

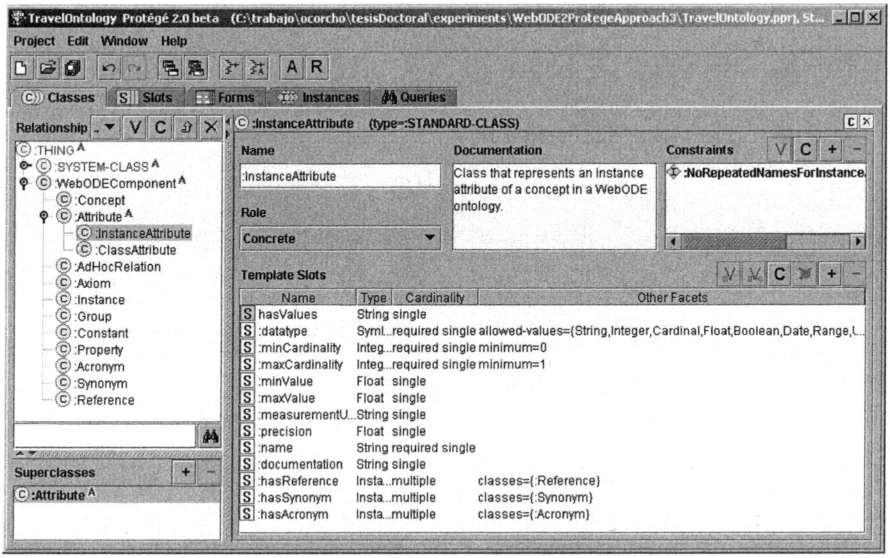

Figure 4.7. WebODE KR ontology modeled in Protégé-2000.

Once this KR ontology has been created in Protégé-2000, the following step consists in transforming the WebODE domain ontology components into instances of the classes and slots of the KR ontology already created. Therefore, the concepts of the original ontology are transformed into instances of the class *:Concept*; its instance attributes are transformed into instances of the class *:InstanceAttribute* and these instances attached to the corresponding instance of *:Concept* with the *:hasAttribute* slot, etc.

Figure 4.8 shows how all the concepts from the source ontology have been transformed into instances of the Protégé-2000 class *:Concept*, and illustrates the details of the concept `accommodation`, with its documentation, the classes of which it is a subclass, etc. As explained above, the main drawback of this approach concerns the pragmatic preservation. In this example, Protégé-2000 users (be them humans or other information systems) will not be able to use the resulting ontology easily. For instance, not even the class taxonomy of the original ontology is shown in Protégé-2000.

Following this approach the inverse transformation (from the ontology generated in Protégé-2000 back to WebODE) is also a simple task. It is not necessary to create any KR ontology in WebODE, since the translation system will back-transform the ontology into the WebODE standard knowledge model. Then, the transformation process would consist again in executing mappings at the lexical and syntax layers.

In case the source format was Protégé-2000 and we wanted to create ontology translation systems to WebODE, and from WebODE to Protégé-2000, the process required is similar to the one already explained in this section. First, the Protégé-2000 KR ontology can be created in WebODE by means of WebODE concepts, instance and class attributes, relations, and formal axioms. Then, the lexical and syntax mappings between Protégé-2000 and the Protégé-2000 KR ontology in WebODE are executed. Finally, to obtain the source ontology back again, new transformations at the lexical and syntax layers must be proposed between the Protégé-2000 KR ontology in WebODE and Protégé-2000.

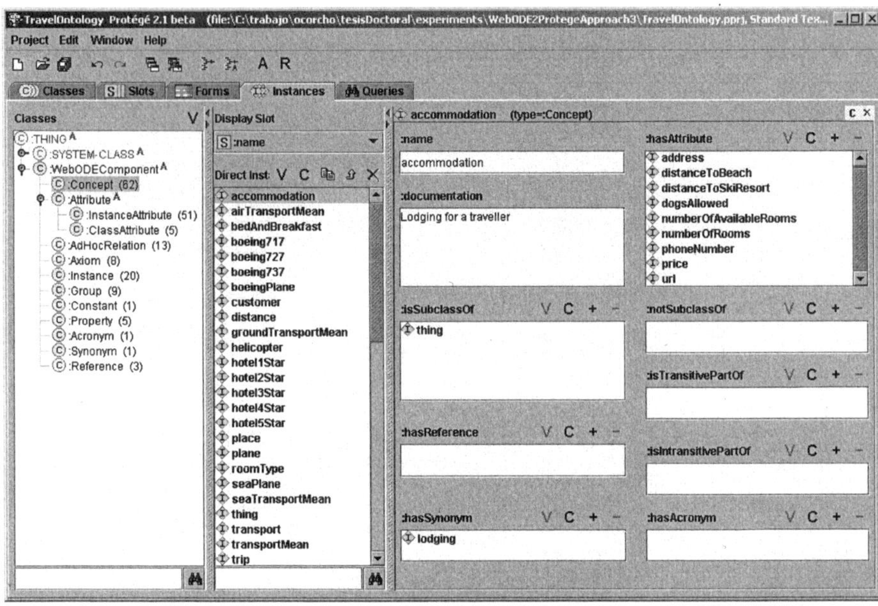

Figure 4.8. Result of a direct translation from WebODE to Protégé-2000 as an instantiation of the WebODE KR ontology.

4.3.3 Direct Translation with the Necessary Additional Components of the Source KR Ontology Only

This approach proposes to transform as much knowledge as possible using the components of the target format's standard knowledge model (as described in section 4.3.1), so that the knowledge transformed can be easily understood and dealt with by human users and applications. Besides, it proposes to manage those pieces of knowledge that have not been transformed, so that they can be recovered in case the ontology is back-transformed (as described in section 4.3.2). This proposal avoids mixing the domain ontology components transformed with the knowledge modeling components used for semantic preservation.

To achieve this twofold objective, this approach proposes to implement part of the source format's KR ontology in the target format, by means of meta-knowledge (which is usually expressed with metaclasses, annotation properties, etc.). The KR ontology implemented contains only the ontology components that cannot be represented directly in the standard knowledge model of the target format, so that these components are only used in case some knowledge of the original ontology cannot be directly transformed into the target format.

In summary, according to this approach the translation of an ontology consists in performing the following steps:

1. To create part of the KR ontology of the source format in the target format, by means of meta-knowledge. This part of the KR ontology models the knowledge modeling components of the source format that have not a direct correspondence with the knowledge modeling components of the target format. Meta-knowledge is usually represented by means of metaclasses (as described by [Dahchour et al., 2001], one of the applications of metaclasses is to define formalisms or development methods within another system). However, this does not prevent us from using other elements, such as annotations (like OWL annotation properties), structured natural language documentations, etc.

2. To transform the component of the original ontology to its corresponding components in the target format whenever there is a direct correspondence between the source format's ontology components and the target format's ones.
3. To transform all the knowledge not transformed in step 2, according to the partial KR ontology created in the first step.

This approach requires that the target format provides some means of representing fragments of KR ontologies in such a way that the domain ontology components transformed are not mixed with the knowledge modeling components used for semantic preservation. Thus we will preserve most of the semantics and pragmatics of the ontology transformed.

Some target formats, such as the ontology tools Protégé-2000 and WebODE, and the ontology markup languages RDF(S) and OWL, provide interesting possibilities for implementing this approach, as described below:

- Protégé-2000 allows representing metaclasses. Metaclasses can be used to create the additional knowledge modeling components needed so that the semantics can be preserved in the transformation. Besides, the Protégé-2000 user interface can be easily configured to hide the additional KR ontology components both from the class taxonomy of the ontology and from the forms used to created domain ontology components. This is useful to preserve the ontology pragmatics in the transformation, because the domain ontology components are not mixed with the other components used for semantic preservation.
- WebODE allows representing metaclasses, as shown in [Fernández-López and Gómez-Pérez, 2002], and importing components from other ontologies. These KR features allow creating two parallel versions of the same ontology, one with the knowledge directly transformed into the standard knowledge model of WebODE, and the other one with the additional knowledge that cannot be transformed directly. In this way, the domain ontology components are not mixed with the other components used for semantic preservation.
- OWL permits attaching annotation properties to any ontology component. Annotation properties do not affect the semantics of the ontology transformed, and can be used to store any extra knowledge that cannot be represented in the standard knowledge model of the language. Additionally, OWL Full allows representing metaclasses.
- RDF(S) allows representing metaclasses, which have the advantages already commented above.

With regard to the number of translation systems needed to perform cyclic transformations, this approach has the same drawbacks than the approach presented in section 4.3.2: it doubles its normal number. However, there is a difference with respect to that approach. If no specific translation system is developed from the language L2 to L1, but just a general one that uses approaches presented in sections 4.2 or 4.3.1, part of the ontology will be at least transformed, while in the previous approach the transformation could not be done at all.

4.3.3.1 Practical Example: from WebODE to Protégé-2000, and vice versa

To illustrate the ontology translation approach presented in this section, we have implemented another ontology translation system between WebODE and Protégé-2000, and vice versa. The objective of this translation system is to reuse as much as possible the standard knowledge model of Protégé-2000, so that the resulting ontology is easy to understand by Protégé-2000 users (either human users or systems), and use the extensibility facilities provided by Protégé-2000 to maintain the rest of knowledge that cannot be directly translated.

Therefore, we have created part of the WebODE KR ontology in Protégé-2000, as shown in figure 4.9, by extending the Protégé-2000 standard metamodel. The following metaclasses have been created: *:WebODEConcept*, *:WebODESlot*, *:WebODEAttribute*, *:WebODEAdHocRelation*, *:WebODEPredefinedSlots*, and *:WebODEPredefinedFacet*. Besides, the following classes have been defined as subclasses of the class *:PAL-CONSTRAINT*, which is used to generate all the PAL constraints in Protégé-2000: *:WebODEDisjointConstraint*, *:WebODEAxiom*, and *:WebODEPropertyConstraint*. Furthermore, subclasses of the predefined class *:THING* have been used to represent some other components: *:WebODEReference*, *:WebODESynonym*, *:WebODEAbbreviation*, *:WebODEConstant*, and *:WebODEProperty*.

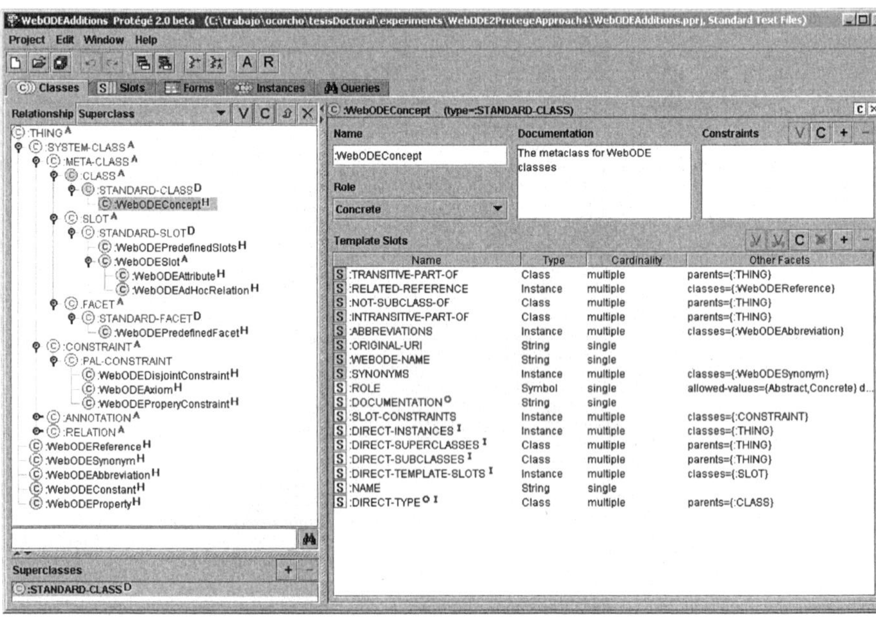

Figure 4.9. Partial WebODE KR ontology represented in Protégé-2000 mainly by means of metaclasses.

The figure shows the details of the metaclass *:WebODEConcept*, which extends the metaclass *:STANDARD-CLASS*, used by default for creating Protégé-2000 classes. The extension consists of some new WebODE specific slots that can store class information not represented in the standard knowledge model of Protégé-2000, such as transitive and intransitive parts of, not subclass of, and bibliographic references, abbreviations, and synonyms. Besides, two other slots are attached to this metaclass; these slots are used also to ensure that in cyclic transformations the original ontology can be recovered: the original URI of the concept in WebODE and its original name, since the class name may have suffered from lexical transformations in the transformation process to Protégé-2000. The rest of information reuses the standard slots for standard classes in Protégé-2000.

This ontology is created as a separate ontology, which is imported by every ontology that results from the application of the ontology translation system created. This translation system works as follows:

- First, it transforms into Protégé-2000 all the WebODE ontology components that have a direct representation in the standard knowledge model of Protégé-2000.
- Second, it transforms the rest of the WebODE ontology components that have not a direct representation in the previous knowledge model. This transformation consists in creating instances of the WebODE KR ontology described above, preserving the knowledge that could have been lost in the translation when the ontology is back-transformed into WebODE.

Figure 4.10 shows a screenshot of the travel ontology translated with this approach. In this example, the metaclass *:WebODEConcept* has a subclass `hotelTypes`, which is consequently another metaclass, used as the metaclass for the classes `hotel1Star`, `hotel2Star`, `hotel3Star`, `hotel4Star`, and `hotel5Star`, as they all have an own slot `numberOfStars` whose value is 1, 2, 3, 4, and 5, respectively. The rest of classes in this ontology are instances of the metaclass *:WebODEConcept.*

The figure shows that, in contrast to the solution presented in section 5.3.2, the classes and class taxonomy of the ontology can be easily seen and understood. The figure also shows the details of the class `hotel1Star`, with its template slots and the own slot `numberOfStars`, coming from the instance attribute and class attribute definition of WebODE. There are also other own slots that do not appear commonly in Protégé-2000 ontologies: *:ORIGINAL-URI*, *:WEBODE-NAME*, *:SYNONYMS*, *:ABBREVIATIONS*, etc. These slots are used to include the extra knowledge from WebODE, as we discussed before.

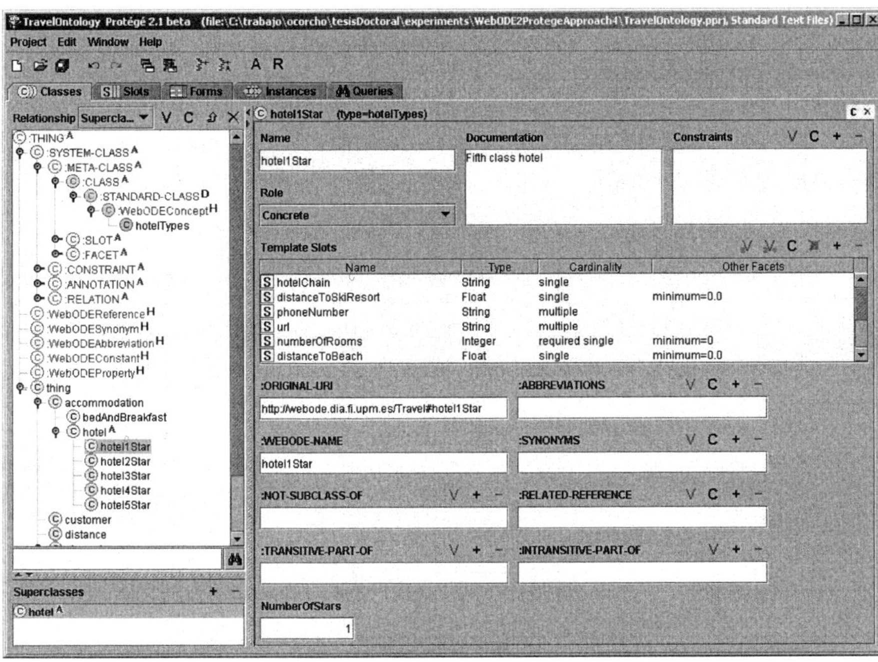

Figure 4.10. Result of a direct translation from WebODE to Protégé-2000 using the standard knowledge model of Protégé-2000 and part of the WebODE KR ontology.

The main drawback of the user interface presented by the previous screenshot is that an end-user who is not acquainted with the knowledge model of WebODE will not be able to understand what the terms *:WebODEReference*, *:WebODESynonym*, etc., mean, since this solution merges the modeling of the domain ontology with the modeling of the KR ontology. We need a last step in this process to ensure that the new components related to the WebODE KR ontology are not shown to Protégé-2000 users.

For this we use the hiding-class functionality provided by Protégé-2000 and remove some components from the forms shown to the users. Consequently, end users do not have to learn how to model ontologies with WebODE and they are shown the ontology with the common modeling conventions provided by Protégé-2000. In the back-transformation into WebODE, this hidden knowledge can be transformed without problems. Figure 4.11 shows the result of configuring Protégé-2000 to hide these classes, and the forms shown for classes.

In conclusion, this proposal meets the two objectives that we had in mind at the beginning of this section: to preserve all the knowledge in the transformation and to allow end users and applications to understand the resulting ontology easily.

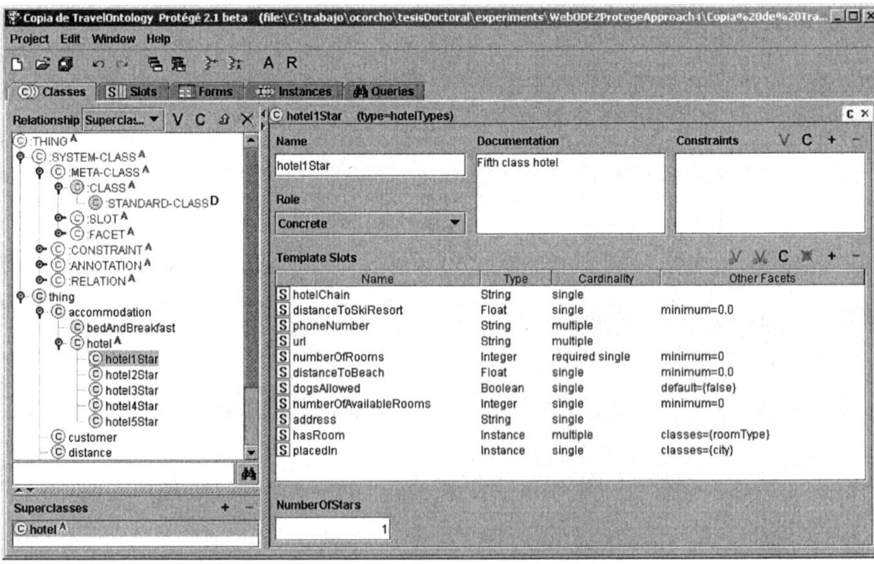

Figure 4.11. Result of a direct translation from WebODE to Protégé-2000 using the Protégé-2000 standard knowledge model and part of the WebODE KR ontology, hiding classes and customizing forms.

Similarly, the same kind of solution can be applied when transforming ontologies from Protégé-2000 into WebODE, as was briefly explained previously: the new components are not shown to WebODE users since they are instances of the WebODE KR ontology and are not accessed directly from the ontology that is result of the transformation. However, the new components are also available for performing the transformation back to Protégé-2000.

The inverse case (translating from Protégé-2000 to WebODE) is equivalent to this one: we should create the Protégé KR ontology in WebODE, as explained in [Fernández-López and Gómez-Pérez, 2002] for the implementation of metaclasses for the ODEClean service, and transform all the components of the Protégé ontology according to it.

Chapter 5
Experimentation

This chapter describes two sets of experiments carried out to evaluate our contributions to the state of the art. The first set consists in creating several ontology translation systems (import and export services) between the WebODE ontology engineering platform and several ontology languages and tools, as well as other general-purpose languages. Some of these translation systems have been used to obtain the layered declarative ontology translation model described in chapter 3, while others have been used to evaluate how such ontology translation model is utilized. The second set of experiments presents results and comparisons of the ontology translation approaches described in chapter 4, from the points of view of semantic and pragmatic preservation.

5.1 Experiments with the Ontology Translation Model

The ontology translation model described in chapter 3 (including the ontology translation method, the distinction of four ontology translation layers, and the ODEDialect set of languages) is derived from our experience in the development of ontology translation systems between the ontology engineering workbench WebODE and different ontology and general-purpose languages, as follows:

- ***Description logic ontology languages***. We have developed WebODE export services to DAML+OIL (based on SHOIQ), OIL (based on SHIQ), and XCARIN (an XML version of the CARIN language, which is based on ALN). Besides, we have developed WebODE import services from the languages DAML+OIL and XCARIN.
- ***Frame-based ontology languages***. We have developed the WebODE export service to FLogic, based on a combination of frames and first order logic.
- ***General-purpose programming languages***. We have developed the WebODE export service to Java, converting the ontology concepts into Java beans.
- ***Markup languages***. We have developed the WebODE export and import services to and from XML, using a DTD that resembles the WebODE knowledge model.

Once the ontology translation model was generated, we evaluated its goodness and refined it by constructing the ontology translation systems between WebODE and RDF(S) (based on a combination of semantic networks and frames), OWL DL (based on description logics), and Protégé-2000 (based on a combination of frames and first order logic), and vice versa. All these translation systems have been successfully integrated as export and import services of the WebODE platform and are currently available for WebODE users. The details of these export and import services are as follows:

- ***WebODE export and import services to and from RDF(S)***. These translation systems have been developed from scratch, following a translation approach mainly driven by pragmatic preservation. We have decided to follow the approach presented in section 4.3.1., that is, perform a direct transformation without any additional components to preserve the semantics of the ontology transformed. We have decided to use this translation approach with the idea of having better interoperability with other ontology tools and ontology-based applications, which would be highly compromised if we used any of the other approaches.

  From a coarse-grained perspective, WebODE concepts are transformed into RDFS classes, WebODE attributes and ad hoc relations are transformed into RDF properties, and WebODE instances are transformed into RDF instances, and vice versa. However, much knowledge is lost in the transformation, such as cardinality constraints in properties, disjoint and exhaustive knowledge in class taxonomies, formal axioms, etc.

- ***WebODE export and import services to and from OWL DL***. These translation systems have been constructed by reusing the export and import services to and from DAML+OIL, and by reusing the RDF export and import services for dealing with instances. The translation approach followed for these export and import services is also driven by pragmatic preservation. As with RDF(S), we have decided to perform a direct transformation without any additional components to preserve the semantics. This decision is made as well to have a better interoperability with other ontology tools and ontology-based applications.

  From a coarse-grained perspective, WebODE concepts are transformed into OWL classes, WebODE attributes into OWL datatype properties, WebODE ad hoc relations into OWL object properties, and WebODE instances into RDF instances, and vice versa. Compared to the RDF(S) translation systems, the amount of knowledge lost in this transformation is much more small, since OWL is much more expressive than RDF(S).

- ***WebODE export and import services to and from Protégé-2000***. These services have been developed from scratch, implemented according to all the ontology translation approaches described in chapter 4. We should be aware that the service currently available has been developed with a hybrid approach, combining direct mappings between components and all the additional components needed in order to preserve knowledge in the transformation, by means of metaclasses and hidden classes (described in section 4.3.3).

Some translation services have been developed in the context of R&D projects: the XCARIN translation services were developed in the context of the EU project MKBEEM (IST-1999-10589), and the DAML+OIL services in the context of the Spanish CICYT project ContentWeb (TIC-2001-2745).

The export and import services to and from RDF(S), OWL DL, and Protégé-2000 have been created in the context of the EU project Esperonto (IST-2001-34373). The objective of this project is to bridge the gap between the current Web and the Semantic Web; that is the reason why the W3C recommendations RDF(S) and OWL DL have been dealt with. Besides, the Protégé-2000 services have been created to allow both tools to exchange their ontologies and to permit using their varied and complementary ontology-based services and applications.

It is important to highlight that the transformations to be done among these formats are quite different to each other. As described above, the WebODE and Protégé-2000 knowledge models are based on a combination of frames and first order logic, OWL DL is based on description logic, and RDF(S) is based on semantic networks, although it provides some basic frame-based KR primitives. Hence the successful application of the ontology translation model for the development of these ontology translation systems shows that the model proposed in this chapter can be used in different contexts and for generating ontology translation systems with different syntaxes and expressiveness capabilities.

All these services are available in the public server of the WebODE ontology engineering workbench[42], and have been used for uploading and implementing ontologies in these languages and in Protégé-2000. We have tested the correct behavior of the export services with all the ontologies available in this server (215 ontologies of different sizes and complexities, and developed by different users), plus the set of synthetic ontologies from the benchmark suite described in [Corcho et al., 2003b]. Besides, 65 RDF(S) ontologies and 55 OWL DL ontologies (of different sizes and complexities, and developed by different users) have been successfully imported in the server by WebODE external users.

5.2 Experiments with Semantic and Pragmatic Preservation in Ontology Translation

The second set of experiments consists in performing cyclic ontology translations between the ontology tools WebODE and Protégé-2000, and then comparing the results obtained at each step according to two parameters: semantic and pragmatic preservation. We have used a representative ontology for performing these experiments: the travel ontology built for the EON2002 experiment, which aimed at showing how different tools can be used to build the same ontology.

In our experiments, we have taken into account the four ontology translation approaches described in chapter 4. For the first translation approach (indirect transformation through common knowledge interchange formats), we have used two ontology markup languages, RDF(S) and OWL DL. The next subsections present the results of each experiment.

5.2.1 Indirect Ontology Translation with RDF(S) as a Common Interchange Format

This experiment consisted in performing a 4-step transformation of the travel ontology: (1) from WebODE to RDF(S), (2) from RDF(S) to Protégé-2000, (3) from Protégé-2000 to RDF(S), and (4) from RDF(S) to WebODE. Both tools already provided export and import services to and from the RDF(S) language. Therefore, no implementation effort has been needed to perform this experiment.

Table 5.1. Summary of the results obtained in the indirect translation between WebODE and Protégé-2000, with RDF(S) as a knowledge interchange format.

	WebODE	**RDF(S) (step 1)**	**Protégé-2000 (step 2)**	**RDF(S) (step 3)**	**WebODE (step 4)**
#concepts	62	62	62	62	62
#subclass of	24	**61**	62	62	62
#disjoint decompositions	6	**0**	0	0	0
#exhaustive decompositions	1	**0**	0	0	0
#partitions	3	**0**	0	0	0
#attributes/relations	69	**43**	43	43	43
#axioms	8	**0**	0	0	0
#constants	1	**0**	0	0	0
#instances	20	20	**22**	22	**20**

[42] *http://webode.dia.fi.upm.es/*

Table 5.1 shows a coarse-grained summary of the results obtained in this experiment. It presents the number of concepts available at each step, the number of subclass-of relationships, of disjoint and exhaustive decompositions of concepts, of concept partitions, of attributes and ad hoc relations, of formal axioms, of constants, and of concept instances. These ontology components will be also the ones used in the rest of experiments. The most representative results are highlighted in bold font, and commented below[43].

As commented in section 5.1, the WebODE export service to RDF(S) transforms only the knowledge that can be represented in the standard knowledge model of this language. Concepts and instances are correctly transformed. The number of attributes and relations decreases because in RDF(S) their scope is global to the ontology, while in WebODE attributes depend on the concept where they are defined. The original ontology contains several attributes and relations with the same name defined in different concepts, and that is the reason why the number of global RDF properties decreases. Furthermore, their cardinality restrictions are lost, since RDF(S) cannot express such knowledge. And in the cases where a property was defined for two different concepts or with two different ranges this information is also lost, since RDF(S) does not allow representing complex property domains and ranges. Besides, formal axioms and constants are lost. Similarly, disjoint and exhaustive knowledge in concept taxonomies is partially lost, and transformed into subclass-of relationships between concepts.

The second step is performed almost correctly by the Protégé-2000 import service from RDF(S). The classes and properties defined in RDF(S) are imported as Protégé-2000 classes and slots, the subclass-of relationships are also transformed correctly (although one extra relationship is created between the root class in the class taxonomy and the predefined Protégé-2000 class *:THING*), and the instances are correctly transformed, though two new instances are created as a result of the values of some properties for some instances, which were resources.

Protégé-2000 gives support to two types of RDF(S) translation: plain RDF(S) and Protégé-2000 specific RDF(S). In the first case, the RDF(S) ontology resulting from the third translation step is similar to the one generated after the first step. The only differences between both ontologies are related to the RDF syntax used in each case, and to the two new instances incorrectly generated. In the second case, the RDF(S) code contains additional tags and attributes that preserve all the knowledge available in the Protégé-2000 ontology. The following piece of code shows such additional information for the RDF property `distanceToSkiResort`, with the Protégé-2000 specific[44] attributes *a:maxCardinality*, *a:minValue*, and *a:range*:

```
<rdf:Property rdf:about="#distanceToSkiResort"
        a:maxCardinality="1"
        a:minValue="0.0"
        a:range="float"
        rdfs:comment="The distance from the hotel to a ski resort"
        rdfs:label="distanceToSkiResort">
   <rdfs:domain rdf:resource="#accommodation"/>
   <rdfs:range rdf:resource="&rdfs;Literal"/>
</rdf:Property>
```

[43] *The results of this experiment are described with more detail in [Corcho et al., 2003a].*

[44] *This example is aimed at showing the RDF(S) code that Protégé-2000 is able to generate. We must note that, as a result of the first transformation step from WebODE to RDF(S), information about cardinalities and minimum values was already lost, and hence does not appear in the Protégé-2000 ontology.*

Finally, the result of the last translation step is a WebODE ontology that contains all the concepts and instances available in the original ontology.

With regard to the rest of the knowledge, the result of the cyclic transformation is as follows: the ontology does not contain the formal axioms and constants that were available initially; the disjoint and exhaustive knowledge in concept taxonomies has been transformed into simple subclass-of relationships between concepts; the properties that had a explicit domain defined are transformed into attributes or relations (depending on whether the range is a datatype or a class) that are attached to the corresponding concept, and in contrast, the properties with no explicit domain defined are transformed into attributes or relations that are attached to the root concept of the taxonomy.

The table and the preceding comments summarize the results related to the preservation of semantics in the translation process. With regard to the preservation of the intended meaning of the ontology, the results obtained are good: the classes and the class taxonomy of the Protégé-2000 ontology are the same as those in the original ontology (except for the disjoint and exhaustive knowledge); and the instances are similar, except for those newly created. With regard to the slots, two different attributes or relations with the same name in WebODE are transformed into a single slot or relation if they have the same range; otherwise they are transformed into different slots or relations, with similar names. Finally, only some term names are different to the original ones, but they are still easily understandable.

5.2.2 Indirect Ontology Translation with OWL DL as a Common Interchange Format

Like the previous experiment, this also consists of four transformation steps, with OWL DL as a common interchange language. Both WebODE and Protégé-2000 provide export and import services to and from OWL DL; hence no implementation effort has been needed to perform this experiment. We must take into account that in the case of Protégé-2000 we had two options: using Protégé-2000 with the OWL plug-in and its own user interface, or using Protégé-2000 with the OWL plug-in but with the general-purpose Protégé-2000 user interface. We have selected the second option, since the general-purpose Protégé-2000 user interface is involved in the rest of experiments, and hence the results obtained here will not be biased by the interchange language used.

Table 5.2 shows a coarse-grained summary of the results obtained in this experiment, with the same knowledge components than in table 5.1, and in which the most representative results are highlighted in bold font.

Table 5.2. Summary of the results obtained in the indirect translation between WebODE and Protégé-2000, with OWL DL as a knowledge interchange format.

	WebODE	**OWL DL (step 1)**	**Protégé-2000 (step 2)**	**OWL DL (step 3)**	**WebODE (step 4)**
#concepts	62	62	62	62	**66**
#subclass of	24	**61**	**62**	62	62
#disjoint decompositions	6	6	**0**	0	0
#exhaustive decomp.	1	1	**0**	0	0
#partitions	3	3	**0**	0	0
#attributes/relations	69	**43**	43	43	43
#axioms	8	**0**	0	0	**4**
#constants	1	**0**	0	0	0
#instances	20	20	20	20	20

In the first transformation step, the figures presented in the table are similar to those obtained in the case of the RDF(S) language, except for the disjoint and exhaustive decompositions, and partitions. Disjoint knowledge is expressed by means of the *owl:disjointWith* primitive between all the pairs of concepts inside the disjoint decomposition or partition. Exhaustive knowledge is expressed by means of the *owl:unionOf* primitive (the superclass is defined as equivalent to the union of all the classes in the exhaustive decomposition or partition). Besides, all the concepts in each decomposition or partition are defined as subclasses of their superclass.

However, there are other differences not shown in the table that are related to the fact that OWL DL is more expressive than RDF(S). For instance, OWL DL can represent property cardinalities, complex domains and ranges in properties, datatype and object properties, etc.

In the second transformation step (from OWL DL to Protégé-2000), the disjoint and exhaustive knowledge in class taxonomies is lost, since it cannot be represented with the standard knowledge model of Protégé-2000, and is not transformed automatically to PAL constraints. The rest of knowledge components are correctly transformed.

Consequently, the OWL DL ontology obtained as a result of the third step (from Protégé-2000 to OWL DL) does not contain the knowledge lost in the previous transformation. However, since Protégé-2000 does not provide specific components in its standard knowledge model for representing this kind of knowledge, this knowledge would never have been transformed.

The most interesting result that appears from the fourth translation process (from OWL DL to WebODE) is the creation of four new classes and formal axioms, which are interrelated. The classes correspond to anonymous classes that come from complex domains of datatype and object properties, while the formal axioms define formally these complex domains. For example, the following formal axiom defines the anonymous class derived from the attribute `numberOfStars`.

```
forall (?x) (OWL_ANONYMOUS_CLASS_3(?x))<->
  ((hotel1Star(?x)) or (hotel2Star(?x)) or (hotel3Star(?x)) or
   (hotel4Star(?x)) or (hotel5Star(?x)))
```

From the pragmatic point of view, the results are similar to those obtained in the previous step. The main differences are related to the transformation of disjoint and exhaustive knowledge in concept taxonomies, as was the case for semantics. Disjoint decompositions are transformed into *rdfs:subClassOf* relationships and *owl:disjointWith* relationships, which are easily understandable. In the case of the back-transformation into WebODE, the most representative aspects appear with the creation of anonymous classes and formal axioms, because unions of classes cannot be easily expressed in frame-based knowledge models. These classes and axioms make the resulting ontology more difficult to understand in WebODE.

5.2.3 Direct Ontology Translation without Additional Semantic Preservation Components

The experiment shown in this section consists of two translation steps: in the first one, the ontology is transformed directly from WebODE into the standard knowledge model of Protégé-2000; in the second step, that ontology is back-transformed from Protégé-2000 into WebODE. The results obtained are summarized in table 5.3. This experiment illustrated section 4.3.1.

The implementation effort for this translation approach is higher than in the previous indirect approaches, because both translation systems had to be developed.

The most relevant aspect to be commented of the first translation step relies on the transformation of disjoint and exhaustive knowledge in concept taxonomies. This knowledge is transformed into *subclass-of* relationships between classes and into PAL constraints, which state either the disjointness between classes, the exhaustiveness of class decompositions or both (the use of PAL constraints was suggested in section 4.3.1). This is why the number of formal axioms in Protégé-2000 is higher than in the original ontology (37 PAL constraints represent this knowledge). The other 8 PAL constraints correspond to the 8 formal axioms defined in the original WebODE ontology.

Table 5.3. Summary of the results obtained in the direct translation between WebODE and Protégé-2000, without additional components for semantic preservation.

	WebODE	**Protégé-2000 (step 1)**	**WebODE (step 2)**
#concepts	62	62	62
#subclass of	24	**61**	**61**
#disjoint decompositions	6	**0**	**0**
#exhaustive decompositions	1	**0**	0
#partitions	3	**0**	**0**
#attributes/relations	69	**43**	**69**
#axioms	8	**45**	**45**
#constants	1	**0**	0
#instances	20	20	20

Other interesting aspects derived from the previous summary are the transformation of WebODE attributes and ad hoc relations into Protégé-2000 slots. These slots are global to the ontology, as occurred with RDF(S) and OWL DL. Thus we obtain the same number of slots than we obtained in the experiments carried out previously.

Minor differences between the original ontology and the one obtained after the transformation are not shown in this summary. For example, the knowledge about precision and measurement units of attributes is lost, since it cannot be represented in the standard knowledge model of Protégé-2000; some datatypes are transformed and others are lost (e.g., XML Schema datatypes); the documentation attached to formal axioms is lost; etc.

In the back-transformation from Protégé-2000 into WebODE, all the original knowledge is obtained back, except the knowledge that was already lost in the first translation step. For example, all the concepts and instances are obtained back, and the attributes and ad hoc relations are correctly distinguished and transformed (moving from 43 slots to 69 attributes and ad hoc relations). The disjoint and exhaustive knowledge is also back-transformed, but instead of using the corresponding WebODE KR primitives, it is transformed back with formal axioms. The reason for this strange behavior is that the translation service from Protégé-2000 to WebODE is not robust enough to identify the formal axioms that deal with disjoint and exhaustive knowledge and convert them into disjoint and exhaustive decompositions or into partitions. Although such an identification can be carried out, it would require a large additional implementation effort only useful in case that the ontology has been transformed into Protégé-2000 from WebODE. Similar situations were described in chapter 4 with KIF, RDF(S), and OWL expressions.

As a consequence of these results, we can say that the translation has preserved most of the semantics of the ontology transformed, except for some components and parts of them. We can state that most of the pragmatics have been preserved in the transformation, except disjoint and exhaustive knowledge in concept taxonomies. This kind of knowledge is back-transformed into formal axioms in WebODE, making it more difficult to understand what they represent in WebODE, where there are other specific primitives to represent that knowledge. Some other differences are related to the fact that the scope of WebODE attributes and ad hoc relations, and of Protégé-2000 slots is distinct. This has been already commented in the previous experiments, since RDF(S) and OWL DL gave also the same treatment to these knowledge components.

5.2.4 Direct Ontology Translation Instantiating the WebODE KR Ontology in Protégé-2000

This experiment consists also of two translation steps: in the first one, the ontology is transformed directly from WebODE into Protégé-2000 by instantiating the WebODE KR ontology that has been implemented in Protégé-2000; in the second step, that ontology is back-transformed from Protégé-2000 into WebODE. The results obtained are summarized in table 5.4. This experiment was shown as a practical example in section 4.3.2.

The implementation effort for this translation approach is lower than in the previous direct approach, since it consists in performing transformations at the lexical and syntax layers, while the previous approaches considered transformations in the four translation layers.

Table 5.4. Summary of the results obtained in the direct translation between WebODE and Protégé-2000, instantiating the WebODE KR ontology represented in Protégé-2000.

	WebODE	**Protégé-2000 (step 1)**	**WebODE (step 2)**
#concepts	62	**14 (predefined)**	62
#subclass of	24	**0**	**24**
#disjoint decompositions	6	**0**	**6**
#exhaustive decompositions	1	**0**	**1**
#partitions	3	**0**	**3**
#attributes/relations	69	**36 (predefined)**	**69**
#axioms	8	**32 (predefined)**	**8**
#constants	1	**0**	**1**
#instances	20	**179**	**20**

As commented in section 4.3.2, the first step to carry out in this approach, before making any ontology transformation, is to create the KR ontology of the source format in the target format. In this specific case, the transformation consists in creating the WebODE KR ontology in Protégé-2000, by means of Protégé-2000 classes and slots. This KR ontology contains 14 classes and 36 slots, together with 32 PAL constraints that express constraints for the instances of such a KR ontology.

The transformation process from WebODE to Protégé-2000 consists in creating instances of the 14 classes, and adding the corresponding values for their slots. Therefore, the Protégé-2000 ontology contains the 179 instances shown in the table.

The back-transformation to WebODE is rather simple, since it consists of lexical and syntax transformations. As a consequence of such a transformation, the ontology obtained back is identical to the original WebODE ontology. Hence, we can state that we have preserved the semantics in the cyclic transformation.

Not only is the semantics preserved in the cyclic transformation, which can be easily proved since the original and the final ontologies are identical. It is also preserved in the Protégé-2000 ontology obtained from the first translation step. The PAL constraints created as part of the WebODE KR ontology implemented in Protégé-2000 ensure that the semantics of the ontology is the same than that of the original WebODE ontology.

Nevertheless, we cannot say the same about pragmatic preservation. Although in cyclic transformations the pragmatics is preserved (again, because we obtain an identical ontology), the ontology obtained in Protégé-2000 is not legible neither by human users nor by most of the ontology-based applications, since every ontology component is represented as an instance. Consequently, this ontology cannot be easily reused, adapted, etc.

Finally, the translation system from Protégé-2000 to WebODE cannot be used for all the ontologies available in Protégé-2000. It can be used only for those ontologies built with WebODE and transformed to Protégé-2000 with the previous translation system.

5.2.5 Direct Ontology Translation with Additional Components

The final experiment consists also of two translation steps: in the first one, the ontology is transformed directly from WebODE to the standard knowledge model of Protégé-2000, using the additional components needed to preserve all the semantics of the original ontology; in the second step, that ontology is back-transformed from Protégé-2000 to WebODE. The results obtained are summarized in table 5.5. This experiment illustrated section 4.3.3.

The implementation effort for this translation approach is higher than in any of the previous approaches. First, we must create the WebODE KR components that are not available in the Protégé-2000 standard knowledge model, and hide them so as not to affect the legibility of the Protégé-2000 ontologies transformed. The transformation consists in mapping the WebODE components to their corresponding Protégé-2000 standard knowledge components, and instantiating the additional components only for expressing the knowledge that cannot be represented in the Protégé-2000 standard knowledge model.

The transformation from Protégé-2000 to WebODE can reuse the translation decisions of the third experiment. Besides, other transformations at the lexical and syntax level have to be performed to translate the additional knowledge that could not be represented in the standard knowledge model of Protégé-2000.

Table 5.5. Summary of the results obtained in the direct translation between WebODE and Protégé-2000, with additional components for semantic preservation.

	WebODE	**Protégé-2000 (step 1)**	**WebODE (step 2)**
#concepts	62	62	62
#subclass of	24	**61**	**24**
#disjoint decompositions	6	**0**	**6**
#exhaustive decompositions	1	**0**	**1**
#partitions	3	**0**	**3**
#attributes/relations	69	**43**	**69**
#axioms	8	**45**	**8**
#constants	1	**0**	**1**
#instances	20	20	20

The results shown in the table summarize the previous comments: Protégé-2000 users (either human users or systems) will obtain a Protégé-2000 ontology with the same 62 classes that were represented in WebODE, 43 slots, some of which are attached to several classes, and 20 instances. Besides, this ontology has 45 PAL constraints, 8 of which come from the 8 WebODE formal axioms, and the rest express the disjoint and exhaustive knowledge in the class taxonomy (although from a graphical point of view, the class taxonomy looks similar). The rest of knowledge needed to preserve all the semantics in the transformation is hidden to Protégé-2000 users, such as the 6 predefined metaclasses and the 9 predefined classes used to preserve semantics in the transformation, as described in section 4.3.3.

With regard to the translation process from Protégé-2000 to WebODE, we obtain an ontology that is identical to the original one. Therefore, we can speak of semantic and pragmatic preservation in cyclic transformations. This approach is the one used for the current WebODE import and export services from and to Protégé-2000.

With regard to the semantics and pragmatics of the ontology obtained in the intermediate step (that is, in Protégé-2000), we must explain that they are also preserved completely, thanks to the direct mappings between components and to the hiding of the additional knowledge transformed to ensure the preservation.

Table 5.6 presents a coarse-grained summary of the results of cyclic transformations with all the approaches described in section 5.2. From this perspective, the table shows that the two approaches that maintain the same components in cyclic transformations are the last ones. The difference between both cases is that from a pragmatic point of view, the last one provides better results, since the ontology in Protégé-2000 is still easy to understand.

Table 5.6. Summary of the results obtained with the different translation approaches.

	Original	**Final**				
		Indirect via RDF(S)	**Indirect via OWL DL**	**Direct without additional components**	**Direct instantiate WebODE KR ontology**	**Direct with additional components**
#concepts	62	62	66	62	62	62
#subclass of	24	62	62	61	24	24
#disjoint decompositions	6	0	0	0	6	6
#exhaustive decompositions	1	0	0	0	1	1
#partitions	3	0	0	0	3	3
#attributes/relations	69	43	43	69	69	69
#axioms	8	0	4	45	8	8
#constants	1	0	0	0	1	1
#instances	20	20	20	20	20	20

Chapter 6
Conclusions and Future Research Problems

This chapter presents the conclusions of our work, focusing on the main advances to the state of the art on ontology translation, namely the proposal of a layered declarative ontology translation model and the analysis of different translation approaches with respect to their semantic and pragmatic preservation properties. In this chapter we identify open research issues in ontology translation between ontology languages and/or tools.

6.1 Conclusions

As described in chapter 2, the **objective of the work** presented in this document has been to advance the state of the art on ontology translation with two main subobjectives:

- The provision of an integrated model to build ontology translation systems, characterized by two main aspects: it takes into account different layers in the translation problems –lexical, syntax, semantic, and pragmatic–, and the translation decisions can be expressed declaratively.
- The analysis of current translation approaches with respect to their semantic and pragmatic preservation properties in the translation processes, especially in the case of cyclic transformations.

We have considered several **research problems** related to our objectives, as follows:

- The lack of consensus about the classification of ontology translation problems. Many classifications exist, with different objectives (semantic interoperability, ontology merge and integration, etc.), but the translation levels inside each classification do not always coincide.
- The lack of integrated methods and techniques that support the complex task of building ontology translation systems. Many of these methods and techniques are applied in an isolated way for some aspects of the ontology translation building process, such as for comparing the source and target formats, for implementing the translation decisions, etc.
- The fact that the existing formal comparison approaches of KR languages rely on the use of translation functions between the source and target formats, but do not specify how these translation functions should be built. Therefore, they are useful only as a starting point for the development of ontology translation systems.
- The fact that the two existing systems that give technological support to the task of building ontology translation systems (OntoMorph and Transmorpher) impose important limits regarding the format of the source and target formats.

- The fact that ontology building methodologies do not describe in detail how knowledge evolves when it is being translated between different formats.
- The lack of detailed studies about the different approaches used so far for ontology translation, and about their impact on the preservation of the semantics and pragmatics of the transformed ontologies, especially in the case of cyclic transformations.

We will now summarize the main **contributions** to the state of the art provided as a result of the work presented in this book.

One of the contributions is related to the **characterization of ontology translation problems in four layers**: lexical, syntax, semantic, and pragmatic. This classification aims at reaching consensus in the characterization of ontology translation problems, since it is based on the work done in other existing theories, such as semiotics, and provides a catalogue of problems that can appear in each layer. Other works only provide examples of transformations to be performed at each layer.

To achieve this objective, in each of the layers we have identified types of problems that must be considered in the translation between two formats. In the lexical and syntax layers, we have identified general types of problems that may appear for any KR format. In the semantic and pragmatic layers, the general types of problems have referred to the cases of transformations between frame-based and description logic based formats, and vice versa.

Another contribution is related to the proposal of ODEDialect as a **declarative language to express transformations**. ODEDialect is innovative in the sense that it provides specific languages for each of the translation layers (ODELex, ODESyntax, and ODESem). Other languages used for developing ontology translation systems (the ones used in OntoMorph and Transmorpher) are general enough to be able to perform all the types of transformations required at all the layers. However, the problems to be solved at each translation layer are different, and consequently we strongly think that they must be solved with special purpose languages, specifically oriented to the types of problems that we aim to solve at each layer.

Besides, ODEDialect improves the support given by the previous languages, which imposed important limits to the types of formats for which ontology translation systems can be created.

The method described in chapter 4 is another important contribution of our work, since it is **the first method specifically created for developing of ontology translation systems**. The use of such method has an important influence on the quality of the ontology translation systems created, because it provides clear guidelines for their development. With this method, the ontology translation decisions implemented by the system are clearly identified, as well as its preservation properties at all translation layers (lexical, syntactic, semantic, and pragmatic).

Furthermore, the iterative lifecycle that the method proposes ensures that the most difficult translation decisions are handled once the developer of the ontology translation system has gathered more knowledge and lessons learned from the development in the previous iterations.

Finally, with regard to our analysis of existing ontology translation approaches, we have also contributed to the current state of the art by **characterizing these approaches according to their preservation properties in the semantic and pragmatic layers**.

During the last decade, common interchange formats were proposed as the optimal alternative to perform translations of ontologies between *n* knowledge representation formats (languages or tools). This consideration was only based on the number of ontology translation systems needed to be able to transform ontologies among *n* KR formats, but not on the preservation properties of the ontology translation process nor on the quality of the translations performed.

As a result of our analysis, we have been able to assess the quality of the transformations performed with these different approaches, with the result that the quality of indirect translations through common interchange formats is rather low in general, compared to the quality of direct translation approaches.

So we have proposed a comparison of direct and indirect approaches according to two parameters: preservation properties of the semantics and pragmatics of the ontology transformed, and required implementation effort of the approach.

Figure 6.1 shows the result of this comparison according to the first set of criteria (preservation properties). The horizontal axis represents the amount of semantic knowledge preserved in the transformation, while the vertical axis represents the amount of pragmatic knowledge preserved in the transformation. We do not aim at providing quantitative measures about the amounts of semantic and pragmatic knowledge preserved in the translation process; we just provide approximate qualitative measures for them. Besides, not all the source and target format pairs behave in the same way with respect to this preservation.

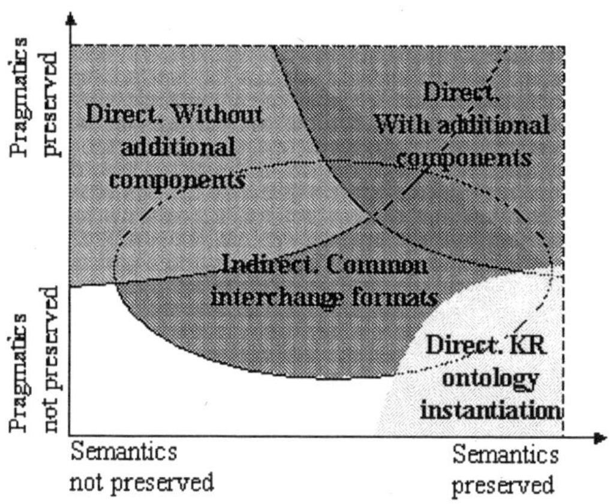

Figure 6.1. Comparison of transformation approaches according to their semantic and pragmatic preservation properties.

As shown in the figure, the direct transformation approaches described in chapter 4 have different behaviors with respect to their preservation properties. The one that ensures maximal preservation properties in the semantic and pragmatic layers is the direct translation where most of the ontology in the source format is transformed to the standard knowledge model of the target format, and additional components and workarounds are only used to preserve the knowledge that could have been lost in the transformation.

With regard to the implementation effort required to carry out each approach, the results are different. The use of common interchange formats does not usually require much implementation effort, since in most cases there are already ontology translation systems implemented for such tasks. With respect to the direct translation approaches, they require more effort: the effort required in the translation without additional components is mainly related to the identification of mappings between the knowledge components of the source and target formats and the implementation of such mappings; the effort required in the direct translation by instantiating the source KR ontology in the target format is mainly devoted to the creation of such KR ontology (the transformation is usually easy, since it has to be done only in the lexical and syntax layers); finally, the hybrid approach requires more effort, because it has to combine the two previous ones.

6.2 Open Research Problems

Even though this document presents important contributions to the current state of the art on ontology translation, there are still some open research problems that have not been taken into account or that have come out as a consequence of the advances to the state of the art proposed. These open research problems, which mainly correspond to the work restrictions already identified in chapter 2, are described below:

- The ontology translation model is aimed at being used to build systems that transform domain ontologies between any pair of ontology languages and/or tools. The model is not specifically designed for other formats that allow representing other types of knowledge, such as knowledge about planning, knowledge about machine learning, etc., nor for other types of ontologies, such as knowledge representation ontologies or upper-level ontologies. Different ontology translation models could be necessary for such specific types of knowledge.
- The ontology translation model does not consider the optimization of the translation process of the system built, neither in terms of space requirements nor in terms of time requirements. This negative aspects are due to the fact that a main requisite for the creation of this model was that it should be easy to create and maintain ontology translation systems, and they should be implemented declaratively. One of the negative impacts of such declarative approaches is that they usually have worse performance (in terms of time and space) than ad hoc solutions.
- The ontology translation model is only aimed at performing translations of full ontologies, and not of part of them. In other words, the model does not consider the possibility of performing incremental translations. These types of translations can be useful when reusing evolving ontologies in a language or tool that is different from the language or tool in which they are available. In some of these cases, an ontology reengineering process must be performed, as described in [Gómez-Pérez and Rojas, 2000], and the ontology transformed is modified after the transformation. Incremental transformations can be used to translate only the parts of the evolving ontology that has changed since the last translation, thus helping to maintain the restructured ontology.
- The three declarative languages that compose ODEDialect (ODELex, ODESyntax, and ODESem) are not expressive enough to represent every possible type of transformation that may appear in any transformation. They only cover the most common types of transformations identified at each layer. If a more complex transformation must be performed, user-defined functions should be used. Additional effort could be devoted to make these languages more expressive so as to cover more types of transformations.
- The analysis of semantic and pragmatic preservation during translation processes described in chapter 4 is restricted to the "representational aspects" of the source and target formats. However, it does not cover other aspects such as the reasoning tractability of the knowledge generated in the target format. This is an important aspect to be considered for many ontology-based applications, which also require that the ontologies transformed are tractable from a reasoning viewpoint.

Appendix I
BNF Grammars of ODELex, ODESyntax, and ODESem

This annex presents the BNF grammars of the three languages that compose ODEDialect: ODELex, ODESyntax, and ODESem. These languages were described in detail in chapter 4.

Notation

The following notation will be used to describe the derivation rules of the ODELex, ODESyntax and ODESem grammars: words in *italics* will be used for non-terminal symbols, words in **bold** font will be used for terminal symbols, alternatives will be represented with the | symbol, optional elements will be enclosed in square brackets **[ ]**, iterations of 0 or more items will be enclosed in braces **{ }**, and ranges of values will be enclosed in parenthesis and separated by hyphens **(-)**.

ODELex Grammar

(1) *ODELexDocument* :: {*comment*} **%%** [*userCode*] **%%** [*declarations*] **%%** [*lexRules*]

(2) *userCode* :: {*comment*} **%(***javaCode***)%**

(3) *declarations* :: {*comment* | *componentDecl* | *overlapDecl*}

(4) *componentDecl* :: *idComponent* [**%transient**] [*scopeDecl*]

(5) *scopeDecl* :: **%scope (** *idScope* {**,** *idScope*} **)**

(6) *idScope* :: *idComponent* | *id*

(7) *overlapDecl* :: **no-overlap (** *idComponent* **,** *idComponent* {**,** *idComponent*} **)**

(8) *lexRules* :: {*lexRule*}

(9) *lexRule* :: *ruleHeader* CR *init* CR *table* CR *repeated* CR *overlap* CR

(10) *ruleHeader* :: **%** *idComponent* **IDENTIFIER** {*idComponent* **IDENTIFIER**}

(11) *init* :: **INIT:{** *javaCode* **}**

(12) *table* :: **TABLE:{** *tableDecl* **}**

(13) *tableDecl* :: **(** *tableColumn* **,** *tableColumn* **)**

(14) *tableColumn* :: **[** *idComponent* **,** *numberPosition* {**,** *numberPosition*}**]**

(15) *numberPosition* :: **%** *number* | **$** *number*

(16) *repeated* :: **REPEATED:{** *transformation* {**,** *transformation*} **}**

(17) *transformation* :: *tablePatternColumn* **==>** {*javaCode* } | **default ==>** {*javaCode* }

(18) *tablePatternColumn* :: **[** *idComponent* **,** *numberPatternPosition*
{**,** *numberPatternPosition*}**]**

(19) *numberPatternPosition* :: **%** *number* | _

(20) *overlap* :: **OVERLAP:{** *javaCode* **}**

(21) *idComponent* :: *idFormat* **.** *id*

(22) *idFormat* :: (**A-Z**){**A-Z**}

(23) *id* :: (**A-Z,a-z**){**a-z,A-Z,0-9**}

(24) *comment* :: /* *textIncludingCR* */ | // *textWithoutCR*

(25) *textIncludingCR* :: {**a-z,A-Z,0-9,CR**}

(26) *textWithoutCR* :: {**a-z,A-Z,0-9**}

(27) *number* :: (**1-9**){**0-9**}

(28) *CR* :: **\n**

ODESyntax Grammar

(1) *ODESyntaxDocument* :: {*comment*} **%%** [*userCode*] **%%** [*declarations*]
%% [*accessDecls*] **%%** [*updateDecls*] **%%** [*datatype*]

(2) *userCode* :: {*comment*} **%(** *javaCode* **)%**

(3) *declarations* :: {*comment* | *namespaceDecl* | *componentDecl* }

(4) *namespaceDecl* :: **%NAMESPACE** *id javaPackage* ;

(5) *componentDecl* :: *idComponent* [*scopeDecl*] **:** *javaClassID* **CR**

(6) *scopeDecl* :: **%scope (** *idComponent* {**,** *idComponent*} **)**

(7) *accessDecls* :: {*accessDecl*}

(8) *accessDecl* :: *header* **CR** [*all* **CR**] [*individual* **CR**] [*information* **CR**]

(9) *header* :: **%** *idComponent* **IDENTIFIER** {*idComponent* **IDENTIFIER**}

(10) *all* :: **ALL:{** *functionDecl* {**;** *functionDecl* } **}**

(11) *individual* :: **INDIVIDUAL:{** *functionDecl* {**;** *functionDecl* } **}**

(12) *functionDecl* :: *number* **:** *id* **(** *parameters* **) :** *javaClassID array*

(13) *parameters* :: **%** *number* { **, %** *number* } | λ

(14) *array* :: **[]** | λ

(15) *information* :: **INFORMATION:{** *informDecl* {**;** *informDecl* } **}**

(16) *informDecl* :: *id* **:** *id* [**(** *parameters* **)**] **:** *javaClassID array*

(17) *updateDecls* :: {*updateDecl*}

(18) *updateDecl* :: *header* **CR** [*create* **CR**] [*remove* **CR**] [*add* **CR**]
[*removeall* **CR**] [*removeindividual* **CR**]

(19) *create* :: **CREATE:{** *createremDecl* {**;** *createremDecl* } **}**

(20) *remove* :: **REMOVE:{** *createremDecl* {**;** *createremDecl* } **}**

(21) *createremDecl* :: *number* **:** *id* **(** *parameters* **)**

(22) *add* :: **ADD:{** *addremDecl* {**;** *addremDecl* } **}**

(23) *removeall* :: **REMOVEALL:{** *addremDecl* {**;** *addremDecl* } **}**

(24) *removeindividual* :: **REMOVEINDIVIDUAL:{** *addremDecl* {**;** *addremDecl* } **}**

(25) *addremDecl* :: *id* **:** *id* **(** *parameters* **)**

(26) *datatype* :: {*datatypeTransf*}

(27) *datatypeTransf* :: **"** *datatypeID* **"** **:** **"** *datatypeID* **"** **;** |
default %1 : (*datatypeID* | **%1** | {*javaCode* })

(28) *idComponent* :: *idFormat* **.** *id*

(29) *idFormat* :: (**A-Z**){**A-Z**}

(30) *id* :: (**A-Z,a-z**){**a-z,A-Z,0-9**}

(31) *comment* :: */* textIncludingCR */* | *// textWithoutCR*

(32) *textIncludingCR* :: {**a-z,A-Z,0-9,CR**}

(33) *textWithoutCR* :: {**a-z,A-Z,0-9**}

(34) *number* :: (**1-9**){**0-9**}

(35) *CR* :: **\n**

(36) *javaClassID* :: **[** *id* **]** *id*

(37) *javaPackage* :: *id* **.** { *id* **.**}

(38) *datatypeID* :: {**a-z,A-Z,0-9,:,/,#**}

ODESem Grammar

(1) *ODESemDocument* :: {*comment*} **%%** [*userCode*] **%%** [*declarations*] **%%** [*semRules*]

(2) *userCode* :: {*comment*} **%(** *javaCode* **)%**

(3) *declarations* :: {*comment* | *ruleDecl* }

(4) *ruleDecl* :: *number* **:** **%** *id* **;**

(5) *semRules* :: {*semRule* | *comment*}

(6) *semRule* :: *header* **CR** *lhs* **-->** **{** *rhs* **}**

(7) *header* :: **%** *id*

(8) *lhs* :: *idComponent id* | **NULL**

(9) *rhs* :: { *create* | *add* | *remove* | *removeall* | *exec* | *ifThen* | *forEach* | *error* | *assign* | *functionCall*} **;**

(10) *assign* :: *id* = { *create* | *functionCall* | *getComponents*}

(11) *functionCall* :: *id* **(** *parameters* **)**

(12) *parameters* :: *id* { **,** *id* } | λ

(13) *ifThen* :: **if (** *condition* **)** [{] *rhs* [}] **else** [{] *rhs* [}]

(14) *condition* :: *javaComparison* | *functionCall*

(15) *forEach* :: **forEach** *id* **IN** *var* [{] *rhs* [}]

(16) *create* :: **CREATE (** *idComponent* **,** *number* **,** *var* {**,** *var*}**)**

(17) *add* :: **ADD (** *id* **,** *id* **,** (*create* | *var* | *getComponents*) **)**

(18) *remove* :: **REMOVE (** *id* **,** *id* **,** *var* **)**

(19) *removeall* :: **REMOVEALL (** *id* **,** *id* **)**

(20) *exec* :: **EXEC (%** *id* **,** *var* **)**

(21) *error* :: **ERROR (** *errorMessage* **)**

(22) *errorMessage* :: **"** *textWithoutCR* **"**

(23) *var* :: *id* | *idComponent*

(24) *getComponents* :: **GETCOMPONENT (** *idComponent* **,** *id* **)** |
GETALLCOMPONENTS (*idComponent* **,** *id* **)**

(25) *idComponent* :: *idFormat* **.** *id*

(26) *idFormat* :: (**A-Z**){**A-Z**}

(27) *id* :: (**A-Z,a-z**){**a-z,A-Z,0-9**}

(28) *comment* :: /* *textIncludingCR* */ | // *textWithoutCR*

(29) *textIncludingCR* :: {**a-z,A-Z,0-9,CR**}

(30) *textWithoutCR* :: {**a-z,A-Z,0-9**}

(31) *number* :: (**1-9**){**0-9**}

(32) *CR* :: **\n**

References

Allen J, Lehrer NB (1992) *Knowledge Representation Specification Language (KRSL) Version 2.0.1.* DARPA/Rome Laboratory Planning and Scheduling Initiative, Reference Manual, ISX Corporation

Arpírez JC, Corcho O, Fernández-López M, Gómez-Pérez A (2001) *WebODE: a scalable ontological engineering workbench.* In: Gil Y, Musen M, Shavlik J (eds) First International Conference on Knowledge Capture (KCAP'01). Victoria, Canada. ACM Press (1-58113-380-4), New York, pp 6-13

Baader F (1996) *A Formal Definition for the Expressive Power of Terminological Knowledge Representation Languages.* Journal of Logic and Computation 6(1):33–54

Baader F, Hollunder B (1991) *KRIS: knowledge representation and inference system.* SIGART Bulletin 2(3):8–14

Baader F, McGuinness D, Nardi D, Patel-Schneider P (2003) *The Description Logic Handbook: Theory, implementation and applications.* Cambridge University Press, Cambridge, United Kingdom

Barley M, Clark P, Williamson K, Woods S (1997) *The neutral representation project.* In: Farquhar A, Grüninger M (eds) AAAI-97 Spring Symposium on Ontological Engineering, Stanford, California. AAAI Press

Bechhofer S, Horrocks I, Goble C, Stevens R (2001a) *OilEd: a reasonable ontology editor for the Semantic Web.* In: Baader F, Brewka G, Eiter T (eds) Joint German/Austrian conference on Artificial Intelligence (KI'01). Vienna, Austria. (Lecture Notes in Artificial Intelligence LNAI 2174) Springer-Verlag, Berlin, Germany, pp 396–408

Bechhofer S, Goble C, Horrocks I (2001b) *DAML+OIL is not enough.* In: Cruz I, Decker S, Euzenat J, McGuinness D (eds) First Semantic Web Working Symposium (SWWS'01). Stanford, California, pp 151–159

Beckett D (2004) *RDF/XML Syntax Specification (Revised).* W3C Recommendation. *http://www.w3.org/TR/rdf-syntax-grammar*

Berk E (1997) *JLex: A lexical analyzer generator for Java,* Technical Report, Department of Computer Science, Princeton University. Latest version available at: http://www.cs.princeton.edu/~appel/modern/java/JLex/current/manual.html

Bernaras A, Laresgoiti I, Corera J (1996) *Building and reusing ontologies for electrical network applications.* In: Wahlster W (ed) European Conference on Artificial Intelligence (ECAI'96). Budapest, Hungary. John Wiley and Sons, Chichester, United Kingdom, pp 298–302

Berners-Lee T (1999) *Weaving the Web: The Original Design and Ultimate Destiny of the World Wide Web by its Inventor.* HarperCollins Publishers, New York

Biron PV, Malhotra A (2001) *XML Schema Part 2: Datatypes.* W3C Recommendation. *http://www.w3.org/TR/xmlschema-2/*

Blázquez M, Fernández-López M, García-Pinar JM, Gómez-Pérez A (1998) *Building Ontologies at the Knowledge Level using the Ontology Design Environment.* In: Gaines BR, Musen MA (eds) 11th International Workshop on Knowledge Acquisition, Modeling and Management (KAW'98). Banff, Canada, SHARE4:1–15

Borgida A (1996) *On the relative expressiveness of description logics and predicate logics*. Artificial Intelligence 82(1-2):353–367

Borgida A, Brachman RJ, McGuinness DL, Resnick LA (1989) *CLASSIC: a structural data model for objects*. In: Clifford J, Lindsay BG, Maier D (eds) ACM SIGMOD International Conference on the Management of Data. Portland, Oregon, pp 58–67

Borst WN (1997) *Construction of Engineering Ontologies*. Centre for Telematica and Information Technology, University of Tweenty. Enschede, The Netherlands

Brachman RJ, Fikes RE, Levesque HJ (1983) *Krypton: A Functional Approach to Knowledge Representation*. IEEE Computer 16(10):67–73

Brachman RJ, Schmolze JG (1985) *An overview of the KL-ONE knowledge representation system*. Cognitive Science 9(2):171–216

Bray T, Paoli J, Sperberg-McQueen CM, Maler E (2000) *Extensible Markup Language (XML) 1.0 (Second Edition)*. W3C Recommendation. *http://www.w3.org/TR/REC-xml*

Brewka G (1987) *The Logic of Inheritance in Frame Systems*. In: McDermott (ed) 10th International Joint Conference on Artificial Intelligence (IJCAI'87), Milan, Italy. Morgan Kaufmann Publishers, San Francisco, California, pp 483–488

Brickley D, Guha RV (2004) *RDF Vocabulary Description Language 1.0: RDF Schema*. W3C Recommendation. *http://www.w3.org/TR/PR-rdf-schema*

Carroll JJ, De Roo J (2003) *OWL Web Ontology Language Test Cases*. W3C Working Draft. *http://www.w3.org/TR/owl-test/*

Chalupsky H (2000) *OntoMorph: a translation system for symbolic knowledge*. In: Cohn AG, Giunchiglia F, Selman B (eds) 7th International Conference on Knowledge Representation and Reasoning (KR'00). Breckenridge, Colorado. Morgan Kaufmann Publishers, San Francisco, California, pp 471–482

Chaudhri VK, Farquhar A, Fikes R, Karp PD, Rice JP (1998) *Open Knowledge Base Connectivity 2.0.3*. Technical Report. *http://www.ai.sri.com/~okbc/okbc-2-0-3.pdf*

Conen W, Klapsing R (2000) *A Logical Interpretation of RDF (discussion paper)*. Linköping Electronic Articles in Computer and Information Science. Journal of Electronic Transactions on Artificial Intelligence 5(13)

Conen W, Klapsing R (2001) *Logical Interpretations of RDFS - A Compatibility Guide*. Working paper. November, 2001. *http://nestroy.wi-inf.uni-essen.de/rdf/new_interpretation/*

Corcho O (2002) *A framework to solve the ontology translation problem*. In: Omelayenko B, Klein M (eds) ECAI'02 Workshop on Knowledge Transformation for the Semantic Web, Lyon, France

Corcho O, Fernández-López M, Gómez-Pérez A, Vicente O (2002) *WebODE: an Integrated Workbench for Ontology Representation, Reasoning and Exchange*. In: Gómez-Pérez A, Benjamins VR (eds) 13th International Conference on Knowledge Engineering and Knowledge Management (EKAW'02). Sigüenza, Spain. (Lecture Notes in Artificial Intelligence LNAI 2473) Springer-Verlag, Berlin, Germany, pp 138–153

Corcho O, García-Castro R, Gómez-Pérez A (2003b) *Towards a benchmark suite for ontology engineering platforms*. In: Volz R, Decker S, Cruz I (eds) ISWC2003 Workshop on Practical and Scalable Semantic Systems (PSSS'2003). Sanibel Island, Florida

Corcho O, Gómez-Pérez A (2000) *A Roadmap to Ontology Specification Languages*. In: Dieng R, Corby O (eds) 12th International Conference in Knowledge Engineering and Knowledge Management (EKAW'00). Juan-Les-Pins, France. Springer-Verlag, Lecture Notes in Artificial Intelligence (LNAI) 1937, Berlin, Germany, pp 80–96

Corcho O, Gómez-Pérez A, Guerrero-Rodríguez DJ, Pérez-Rey D, Ruiz-Cristina A, Sastre-Toral T, Suárez-Figueroa MC (2003a) *Evaluation experiment of ontology tools' interoperability with the WebODE ontology engineering workbench*. In: Sure Y, Corcho O, Angele J (eds) ISWC2003 Workshop on Evaluation of Ontology Tools (EON2003). Sanibel Island, Florida. CEUR Workshop Proceedings 87. Amsterdam, The Netherlands (*http://CEUR-WS.org/Vol-87/*), pp 103-111

Corcho O, Gómez-Pérez A (1999) *Guidelines to Study Differences in Expressiveness between Ontology Specification Languages*. In: 12th Workshop on Knowledge Acquisition, Modeling and Management (KAW'99). Banff, Canada

Dahchour M, Pirotte A, Zimányi E (2001) *Definition and application of metaclasses*. In: Mayr HC, Lazansky J, Quirchmayr G, Vogel P (eds) 12th International Conference on Database and Expert Systems Applications (DEXA'01), Munich, Germany. Springer Verlag Lecture Notes in Computer Science (LNCS) 2113. Berlin, Germany, pp 32–41

Dean M, Schreiber G (2004) *OWL Web Ontology Language Reference*. W3C Recommendation. *http://www.w3.org/TR/owl-ref/*

Decker S, Brickley D, Saarela J, Angele J (1998) *A Query and Inference Service for RDF*. In: Marchiori M (ed) The Query Languages Workshop (QL'98). Boston, Massachusetts. *http://www.w3.org/TandS/QL/QL98/pp/queryservice.html*

Domingue J (1998) *Tadzebao and WebOnto: Discussing, Browsing, and Editing Ontologies on the Web*. In: Gaines BR, Musen MA (eds) 11th International Workshop on Knowledge Acquisition, Modeling and Management (KAW'98). Banff, Canada, KM4:1–20

Euzenat J (2001) *Towards a principled approach to semantic interoperability*. In: Gómez-Pérez A, Grüninger M, Stuckenschmidt H, Uschold M (eds) IJCAI2001 Workshop on Ontologies and Information Sharing, Seattle, Washington

Euzenat J (2002) *An infrastructure for formally ensuring interoperability in a heterogeneous semantic web*. In: Cruz I, Decker S, Euzenat J, McGuinness D (eds) The emerging semantic web, IOS press, Ámsterdam, The Netherlands, pp245-260

Euzenat J, Stuckenschmidt H (2002) *The "family of languages" approach to semantic interoperability*. In: Omelayenko B, Klein M (eds) ECAI'02 Workshop on Knowledge Transformation on the Semantic Web, Lyon, France, pp 93–100

Euzenat J, Stuckenschmidt H (2003) *The 'family of languages' approach to semantic interoperability*. In: Omelayenko B, Klein M (eds) Knowledge transformation for the semantic web, IOS press, Ámsterdam, The Netherlands, pp49-63

Euzenat J, Tardif L (2001) *XML transformation flow processing*. Markup languages: theory and practice 3(3):285–311

Farquhar A, Fikes R, Rice J (1997) *The Ontolingua Server: A Tool for Collaborative Ontology Construction*. International Journal of Human Computer Studies. 46(6):707–727

Fernández-López M, Gómez-Pérez A (2002) *The integration of OntoClean in WebODE*. In: Angele J, Sure Y (eds) EKAW'02 Workshop on Evaluation of Ontology-based Tools (EON2002), Sigüenza, Spain. CEUR Workshop Proceedings 62:38–52. Amsterdam, The Netherlands. *http://CEUR-WS.org/Vol-62/*

Fernández-López M, Gómez-Pérez A, Pazos A, Pazos J (1999) *Building a Chemical Ontology Using Methontology and the Ontology Design Environment*. IEEE Intelligent Systems & their applications 4(1):37–46

Fikes R, McGuinness D (2001) *An Axiomatic Semantics for RDF, RDF Schema, and DAML+OIL*. KSL Technical Report KSL-01-01. Stanford, California. *http://www.w3.org/TR/daml+oil-axioms*

Fillies C (2003) *SemTalk EON2003 Semantic Web Export / Import Interface Test*. In: Sure Y, Corcho O, Angele J (eds) ISWC2003 Workshop on Evaluation of Ontology Tools (EON2003). Sanibel Island, Florida. CEUR Workshop Proceedings 87. Amsterdam, The Netherlands (*http://CEUR-WS.org/Vol-87/*), pp 112-116

Fillies C, Wood-Albrecht G, Weichhardt F (2002) *A Pragmatic Application of the Semantic Web Using SemTalk*. In: WWW2002, Honolulu, Hawaii, ACM 1-5811-449-5/02/0005

Friedman-Hill E (2003) *Jess in Action: Java Rule-Based Systems*. Manning Publications Company, Greenwich, Connecticut

Fulton JA and colleagues (1992) *Technical report on the Semantic Unification Meta-Model: Volume 1 - Semantic unification of static models*. ISO TC184/SC4 WG3 Document N175. ISO/TR 10303-12

Garshol LM (2001) *Topic maps, RDF, DAML, OIL*. In: XML 2001, Orlando, Florida. Available from *http://www.ontopia.net/topicmaps/materials/tmrdfoildaml.html*.

Garshol LM (2003) *Living with topic maps and RDF*. Ontopia technical report. Available from http://www.ontopia.net/topicmaps/materials/tmrdf.html

Genesereth MR (1990) *The Epikit Manual*. Technical Report. Epistemics Inc., Palo Alto, California. *http://logic.stanford.edu/papers/epikit-1.4-manual.ps*

Genesereth MR, Fikes RE (1992) *Knowledge Interchange Format. Version 3.0. Reference Manual*. Technical Report Logic-92-1. Computer Science Department. Stanford University, California, available at *http://meta2.stanford.edu/kif/Hypertext/kif-manual.html*

Gennari JH, Musen MA, Fergerson RW, Grosso WE, Crubézy M, Eriksson H, Noy NF, Tu SW (2003) *The Evolution of Protégé: An Environment for Knowledge-Based Systems Development*. International Journal of Human-Computer Studies 58(1):89–123

Gil Y, Ratnakar V (2002) *A comparison of (semantic) markup languages*. In: Omelayenko B (ed) 15th International FLAIRS Conference, Special Track on Semantic Web, Pensacola, Florida

Ginsberg ML (1991) *Knowledge Interchange Format: the KIF of Death*. AI Magazine 12(3):57–63

Gómez-Pérez A (2001) *Evaluation of Ontologies*. International Journal of Intelligent Systems 16(3):391–409

Gómez-Pérez A (2002) *A Survey on Ontology Tools*, OntoWeb deliverable D1.3. *http://ontoweb.aifb.uni-karlsruhe.de/About/Deliverables/D13_v1-0.zip*

Gómez-Pérez A, Corcho O (2002) *Ontology Languages for the Semantic Web*. IEEE Intelligent Systems & their applications 17(1):54–60

Gómez-Pérez A, Fernández-López M, Corcho O (2003) *Ontological Engineering: with examples from the areas of knowledge management, e-commerce and the Semantic Web*, Springer-Verlag, New York.

Gómez-Pérez A, Juristo N, Montes C, Pazos J (1997) *Ingeniería del Conocimiento*. Centro de Estudios Ramón Areces

Gómez-Pérez A, Rojas MD (1999) *Ontological Reengineering for Reuse*. In: Fensel D, Studer R (eds) 11th European Workshop on Knowledge Acquisition, Modeling and Management (EKAW'99). Dagstuhl Castle, Germany. Springer-Verlag, Lecture Notes in Computer Science (LNCS) 1621, Berlin, Germany, pp 139–156

Gómez-Pérez A, Rojas MD (2000) *Ontological Reengineering and Reuse*. In: Dieng R, Corby O (eds) 12th International Conference in Knowledge Engineering and Knowledge Management (EKAW'00). Juan-Les-Pins, France. Springer-Verlag, Lecture Notes in Artificial Intelligence (LNAI) 1937, Berlin, Germany, pp 139–156

Gruber TR (1992) *Ontolingua: A Mechanism to Support Portable Ontologies*. Technical report KSL-91-66, Knowledge Systems Laboratory, Stanford University, Stanford, California. *ftp://ftp.ksl.stanford.edu/pub/KSL_Reports/KSL-91-66.ps*

Gruber TR (1993a) *A translation approach to portable ontology specification*. Knowledge Acquisition 5(2):199–220

Gruber TR (1993b) *Toward principles for the design of ontologies used for knowledge sharing*. In: Guarino N, Poli R (eds) International Workshop on Formal Ontology in Conceptual Analysis and Knowledge Representation. Padova, Italy. Kluwer Academic Publishers, Deventer, The Netherlands. *http://citeseer.nj.nec.com/gruber93toward.html*

Guarino N (1998) *Formal Ontology in Information Systems*. In: Guarino N (ed) 1st International Conference on Formal Ontology in Information Systems (FOIS'98). Trento, Italy. IOS Press, Amsterdam, pp 3–15

Guarino N, Giaretta P (1995) *Ontologies and Knowledge Bases: Towards a Terminological Clarification*. In: Mars N (ed) Towards Very Large Knowledge Bases: Knowledge Building and Knowledge Sharing (KBKS'95). University of Twente, Enschede, The Netherlands. IOS Press, Amsterdam, The Netherlands, pp 25–32

Haarslev V, Möller R (2001) *Description of the RACER System and its Applications*. In: Goble CA, McGuinness DL, Möller R, Patel-Schneider PF (eds) International Workshop on Description Logics (DL'01). Stanford University, California. CEUR Workshop Proceedings 49:132–141. Amsterdam, The Netherlands (*http://CEUR-WS.org/Vol-49/*)

Hayes P (2004) *RDF Semantics*. W3C Recommendation. *http://www.w3.org/TR/rdf-mt/*

Hermenegildo M, Bueno F, Cabeza D, Carro M, García M, López P, Puebla G (2000) *The Ciao Logic Programming Environment*. In: Lloyd JW, Dahl V, Furbach U, Kerber M, Lau K, Palamidessi C, Pereira LM, Sagiv Y, Stuckey PJ (eds) International Conference on Computational Logic (CL'00). London, United Kingdom. Lecture Notes in Computer Science (LNCS) 1861.

Horrocks I, Fensel D, Harmelen F, Decker S, Erdmann M, Klein M (2000) *OIL in a Nutshell*. In: Dieng R, Corby O (eds) 12th International Conference in Knowledge Engineering and Knowledge Management (EKAW'00). Juan-Les-Pins, France. Springer-Verlag, Lecture Notes in Artificial Intelligence (LNAI) 1937, Berlin, Germany, pp 1–16

Horrocks I, Sattler U, Tobies S (1999) *Practical reasoning for expressive description logics*. In: Ganzinger H, McAllester D, Voronkov A (eds) 6th International Conference on Logic for Programming and Automated Reasoning (LPAR'99). Tbilisi, Georgia. Springer-Verlag, Lecture Notes in Artificial Intelligence (LNAI) 1705, pp 161–180

Horrocks I, van Harmelen F (eds) (2001) *Reference Description of the DAML+OIL (March 2001) Ontology Markup Language*. Technical report. *http://www.daml.org/2001/03/reference.html*

Hudson SE (1999) *Cup's User Manual*, Technical Report, Graphic Visualization and Usability Center, Georgia Institute of Technology. Latest version available at: http://www.cs.princeton.edu/~appel/modern/java/CUP/manual.htm

IEEE (1996) *IEEE Standard for Developing Software Life Cycle Processes*. IEEE Computer Society. New York. IEEE Std 1074-1995

IEEE (1999) *IEEE Guide for Information Technology-Software Reuse*. IEEE Computer Society. New York. IEEE Std. 1430-1996

Isaac A, Troncy R, Malaise V (2003) *Using XSLT for Interoperability: DOE and The Travelling Domain Experiment*. In: Sure Y, Corcho O, Angele J (eds) ISWC2003 Workshop on Evaluation of Ontology Tools (EON2003). Sanibel Island, Florida. CEUR Workshop Proceedings 87. Amsterdam, The Netherlands (*http://CEUR-WS.org/Vol-87/*), pp 92-102

Johnson SC (1975) *Yacc: Yet Another Compiler Compiler*, Computing Science Technical Report No. 32, Bell Laboratories, Murray Hill, New Jersey

Karp PD, Chaudhri V, Thomere J (1999) *XOL: An XML-Based Ontology Exchange Language*. Version 0.3. Technical Report. *http://www.ai.sri.com/~pkarp/xol/xol.html*

Karvounarakis G, Christophides V (2002) *The RQL v1.5 User Manual*. Technical Report, 2002. *http://139.91.183.30:9090/RDF/RQL/Manual.html*

Kifer M, Lausen G, Wu J (1995) *Logical Foundations of Object-Oriented and Frame-Based Languages*. Journal of the ACM 42(4):741–843

Klein M (2001) *Combining and relating ontologies: an analysis of problems and solutions*. In: Gómez-Pérez A, Grüninger M, Stuckenschmidt H, Uschold M (eds) IJCAI2001 Workshop on Ontologies and Information Sharing, Seattle, Washington

Knublauch H (2003) *Editing Semantic Web Content with Protégé: the OWL Plugin*. 6th Protégé workshop. Manchester, United Kingdom

Larman C (2001) *Applying UML and patterns: an introduction to object-oriented analysis and design and the Unified Process*, Prentice Hall PTR

Lassila O, McGuinness D (2001) *The Role of Frame-Based Representation on the Semantic Web*. Technical Report KSL-01-02. Knowledge Systems Laboratory. Stanford University. Stanford, California

Lassila O, Swick R (1999) *Resource Description Framework (RDF) Model and Syntax Specification*. W3C Recommendation. *http://www.w3.org/TR/REC-rdf-syntax/*

Lee J, Grunninger M, Jin Y, Malone T, Tate A, Yost G, and other members of the PIF Working Group (1998) *The PIF Process Interchange Format and Framework Version 1.2*. The Knowledge Engineering Review 13(1):91–120

Lenat DB, Guha RV (1990) *Building Large Knowledge-based Systems: Representation and Inference in the Cyc Project*. Addison-Wesley, Boston, Massachusetts

Lesk ME (1975) *Lex - A Lexical Analyzer Generator*, Computing Science Technical Report No. 39, Bell Laboratories, Murray Hill, New Jersey

Levine R, Mason T, Brown D (1992) *Lex & Yacc*, O'Reilly & Associates, second edition Sebastopol, Canada

Levy AY, Rousset MC (1998) *CARIN: A Representation Language Combining Horn rules and Description Logics*. Artificial Intelligence Journal 104(1-2): 165–209

Luke S, Heflin J (2000) *SHOE 1.01. Proposed Specification*. Technical Report. Parallel Understanding Systems Group. Department of Computer Science. University of Maryland. *http://www.cs.umd.edu/projects/plus/SHOE/spec1.01.htm*

MacGregor R (2001) *Inside the LOOM classifier*. SIGART Bulletin 2(3):88–92

Maedche A, Motik B, Stojanovic L, Studer R, Volz R (2003) *Ontologies for Enterprise Knowledge Management*. IEEE Intelligent Systems 18(2):26–33

Maedche A, Schnurr HP, Staab S, Studer R (2000) *Representation Language-Neutral Modeling of Ontologies*. In: Frank U (eds) German Workshop "Modellierung 2000". Koblenz, Germany, pp 128–144

Manzano M (1999) *Model Theory*, Oxford University Press, Oxford, United Kingdom

METRICA v.3. *MÉTRICA versión 3. Metodología de planificación, desarrollo y mantenimiento de sistemas de información*. Technical Report, Ministerio para las Administraciones Publicas, Spain. http://www.map.es/csi/metrica3.

Morik K, Causse K, Boswell R (1991) *A Common Knowledge Representation Integrating Learning Tools*. In: Michalski RS, Tecuci G (eds) First International Workshop on Multistrategy Learning, Harpers Ferry, WV, pp 81–96.

Morris CW (1938) *Foundations of the theory of signs*. In: Neurath O, Carnap R, Morris CW (eds) International encyclopedia of unified science. Chicago University Press [reprinted in C W Morris 1971 *Writings on the theory of signs*. Mouton, The Hague]

Motta E (1999) *Reusable Components for Knowledge Modeling: Principles and Case Studies in Parametric Design*. IOS Press. Amsterdam, The Netherlands

Mowbray TJ, Zahavi R (1995) *The essential CORBA: System Integration Using Distributed Objects*. John Wiley & Sons and Object Management Group, Chichester, United Kingdom

Musen MA (1989) *Automated support for building and extending expert models*. Machine Learning 4:347–376

NCITS (1998) *Draft proposed American National standard for Knowledge Interchange Format*. National Committee for Information Technology Standards, Technical Committee T2 (Information Interchange and Interpretation). *http://logic.stanford.edu/kif/dpans.html*

Neches R, Fikes RE, Finin T, Gruber TR, Senator T, Swartout WR (1991) *Enabling technology for knowledge sharing*. AI Magazine 12(3):36–56

Newell A (1982) *The Knowledge Level*. Artificial Intelligence 18(1):87–127

Ny NF, Fergerson RW, Musen MA (2000) *The knowledge model of Protege-2000: Combining interoperability and flexibility*. In: Dieng R, Corby O (eds) 12th International Conference in Knowledge Engineering and Knowledge Management (EKAW'00). Juan-Les-Pins, France. (Lecture Notes in Artificial Intelligence LNAI 1937) Springer-Verlag, Berlin, Germany, pp 17–32

Noy NF, Sintek M, Decker S, Crubézy M, Fergerson RW, Musen MA (2001) *Creating Semantic Web contents with Protégé-2000*. IEEE Intelligent Systems 16(2):60–71

Patel-Schneider PF, Hayes P, Horrocks I (2004) *OWL Web Ontology Language Semantics and Abstract Syntax*. W3C Recommendation. *http://www.w3.org/TR/owl-semantics/*

Polikoff I, Allemang D (2003) *TopQuadrant Technology Briefing. Semantic Technology v1.1*. TopQuadrant technical report, available at http://www.topquadrant.com/documents/TQ03_Semantic_Technology_Briefing.pdf

Raggett D, Le Hors A, Jacobs I (1999) *HTML 4.01 Specification*. W3C Recommendation. *http://www.w3.org/TR/html401/*

Raschid L, Vidal ME (1996) *A KIF for Multiple F-Logic databases*, Technical report, Institute for Advanced Computer Studies University of Maryland, ftp://ftp.umiacs.umd.edu/pub/ONRrept/cikm-kif96.ps

Russell S, Norvig P (1995) *Artificial Intelligence: A Modern Approach*. Englewood Cliffs, New Jersey

Schreiber ATh, Wielinga BJ, Jansweijer W (1995) *The KACTUS View on the 'O' World.* In Skuce D (ed) IJCAI95 Workshop on Basic Ontological Issues in Knowledge Sharing, pp 15.1–15.10

Schreiber G, Akkermans H, Anjewierden A, de Hoog R, Shadbolt N, van de Velde W, Wielinga B (1999) *Knowledge engineering and management. The CommonKADS Methodology.* MIT press, Cambridge, Massachusetts

Sintek M, Decker S (2001) *TRIPLE - An RDF Query, Inference, and Transformation Language.* In: Seipel D (ed) Deductive Databases and Knowledge Management (DDLP'01). Tokyo, Japan, pp 364–378

Spiby P (1992) *EXPRESS language for product descriptions.* ISO 10303 Industrial Automation Systems - Product Data Representation and Exchange - Part 11: Description Methods: The EXPRESS Language Reference Manual. ISO DIS 10303-11:1992(E)

Staab S, Schnurr HP, Studer R, Sure Y (2001) *Knowledge Processes and Ontologies.* IEEE Intelligent Systems 16(1):26–34

Stanley MT (1986) *CML: a knowledge representation language with application to requirements modeling.* MS thesis. University of Toronto, Toronto, Canada.

Stuckenschmidt H (2003) *Ontology-Based Information Sharing in Weakly-Structure Environments*, PhD Thesis, Faculty of Sciences, Vrije Universiteit Ámsterdam

Studer R, Benjamins VR, Fensel D (1998) *Knowledge Engineering: Principles and Methods.* IEEE Transactions on Data and Knowledge Engineering 25(1-2):161–197

Sure Y, Corcho O, Angele J (2003) *Proceedings of the EON2003 Workshop on Evaluation of Ontology Tools (EON2003)*, Sanibel Island, Florida. CEUR Workshop Proceedings 87. Amsterdam, The Netherlands (*http://CEUR-WS.org/Vol-87/*)

Sure Y, Staab S, Angele J (2002) *OntoEdit: Guiding Ontology Development by Methodology and Inferencing.* In: Meersman R, Tari Z (eds) Confederated International Conferences CoopIS, DOA and ODBASE 2002, University of California, Irvine. (Lecture Notes in Computer Science LNCS 2519) Springer-Verlag, Berlin, Germany, pp 1205–1222

Swartout B, Ramesh P, Knight K, Russ T (1997) *Toward Distributed Use of Large-Scale Ontologies.* In: Farquhar A, Gruninger M, Gómez-Pérez A, Uschold M, van der Vet P (eds) AAAI'97 Spring Symposium on Ontological Engineering. Stanford University, California, pp 138–148

Uschold M, Grüninger M (1996) *Ontologies: Principles, Methods and Applications.* Knowledge Engineering Review 11(2):93–155

Uschold M, Jasper R (1999) *A Framework for Understanding and Classifying Ontology Applications.* In: Benjamins VR (ed) IJCAI'99 Workshop on Ontology and Problem Solving Methods: Lessons Learned and Future Trends. Stockholm, Sweden. CEUR Workshop Proceedings 18:11.1–11.12. Amsterdam, The Netherlands (*http://CEUR-WS.org/Vol-18/*)

Valente A, Russ T, MacGregor R, Swartout W (1999) *Building and (Re)Using an Ontology of Air Campaign Planning.* IEEE Intelligent Systems & their applications 14(1):27–36

van Harmelen F, Patel-Schneider PF, Horrocks I (2001) *A Model-Theoretic Semantics for DAML+OIL (March 2001).* Technical Report. *http://www.daml.org/2001/03/model-theoretic-semantics.html*

Welty C, Guarino N (2001) *Supporting Ontological Analysis of Taxonomic Relationships.* Data and Knowledge Engineering 39(1):51–74

Woods WA (1983) *What's important about knowledge representation.* IEEE Computer, 16(10)

Subject Index